Life

RECONSTRUCTED

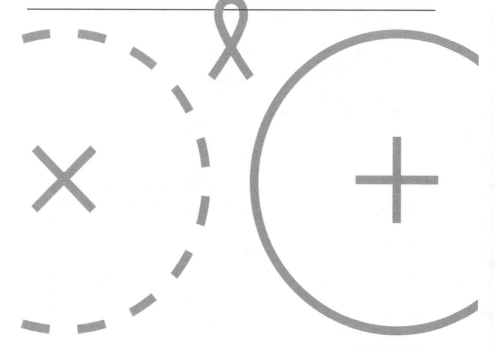

Published by Familius LLC, www.familius.com
1254 Commerce Way, Sanger, CA 93657

Familius books are available at special discounts for bulk purchases, whether for sales promotions or for family or corporate use. For more information, contact Familius Sales at 559-876-2170 or email orders@familius.com.

Library of Congress Control Number: 2021938986

Print ISBN 9781641705677
Ebook ISBN 9781641706278

Printed in the United States of America

Edited by Laurie Duersch and Sarah Echard
Cover design by Derek George
Book design by Maggie Wickes

10 9 8 7 6 5 4 3 2 1

First Edition

Praise for *Life Reconstructed*

"In astonishing honesty and clear detail, Kim Harms takes the reader on an intensely personal journey. She shares experiences and emotions related to her breast reconstructions and illustrates the importance of honorable friends and family, her steadfast faith, and a loving partner."

—**Jacqueline Wagner, RN, OCN, CBCN, Marshfield Clinic Health System**

"Everyone needs to read this book to educate themselves; not just those who receive a cancer diagnosis . . . EVERYONE! Cancer touches us all in some way. Kim Harms does an excellent job of informing, educating, and offering tips, techniques, and resources. As a mental health therapist and five-year cancer survivor, I am excited to see how much research and valuable information she has packed into this book. It is a MUST read."

—**Kathy Thompson, ATR, LPC, CADC, NCC, licensed professional counselor and breast cancer survivor**

"Kim Harms has penned a hopeful and helpful book to help women navigating breast cancer. When I first was diagnosed with breast cancer, I tried to read information and books to help me in my treatment decision process. Looking back, I didn't have a resource to help me navigate the complicated decisions and implications of breast reconstruction. I'm so glad Life Reconstructed is available now. Kim's story and the many resources she cites gives this book both warmth and substance."

—**Vivian Mabuni, national speaker and author of *Warrior in Pink* and *Open Hands, Willing Heart***

"As a general surgeon, I want my patients to be empowered with knowledge that will help them make the best-informed decisions about treatment options and set them up for success in the aftermath of life-altering diagnoses and surgeries. In the realm of breast cancer, mastectomy, and reconstruction, Kim Harms has created an incredible resource for women and for those who love them. Speaking very honestly from personal experience, while also gleaning from the experience of others, Harm's words are not only empowering but also offer hope."

—Heidi J. Haun, MD, FACS,
Baptist Medical Centre, Nalerigu, Ghana

"In Life Reconstructed, Kim Harms takes breast reconstruction— an event far too many women experience—and compassionately guides readers through the process. She skillfully explains the technical issues involved, but also dives into the reactions and emotions that inevitably add to the confusion of breast reconstruction. As a breast cancer plus double mastectomy survivor myself, Life Reconstructed would have been a sweet companion as I traveled through my own journey. May Kim Harm's words bless and comfort many women."

—Katherine James, breast cancer survivor
and author of *Can You See Anything Now* and *A Prayer for Orion*

"Women undergoing mastectomies and breast reconstruction need a shoulder to lean on and trustworthy guidance. Cancer survivor Kim Harms delivers that—and so much more. Life Reconstructed provides vital information, vulnerable stories, and perhaps most importantly, an abundance of compassion."

—Dorothy Littell Greco,
author of *Marriage in the Middle* and *Making Marriage Beautiful*

Life

RECONSTRUCTED

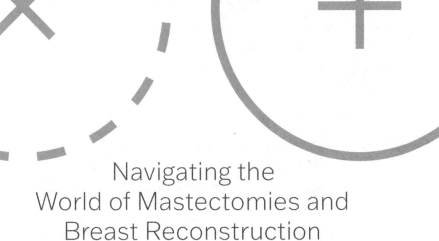

Navigating the
World of Mastectomies and
Breast Reconstruction

KIM HARMS

Contents

In memory of Jodi Lynn Brown

"But those who hope in the Lord will renew their strength. They will soar on wings like eagles; they will run and not grow weary, they will walk and not be faint."
—Isaiah 40:31 (NIV)

1969–2019

Acknowledgments

To Mom and Dad, somehow you ended up with one artist and one writer and you've never told either of us to go get "real" jobs.

To Corey, you are my favorite. You've loved me at my worst, and you believed I could write a book before I believed it myself.

To Carter, Owen, and Lewis, you guys bring me great happiness. My sincerest apologies that when your friends ask you what your mom's book is about, you have to answer "boobs."

To my agent Karen Neumair, thank you for believing in me and for working so hard to get my book proposal into the hands of the perfect publisher.

To Christopher Robbins at Familius Publishing, thank you for taking a risk on this newbie writer.

To Laurie Duersch, my editor, I would work with you a million times. I can't imagine a better first-time book editing experience.

To Jolene Philo, my mentor and friend, I wouldn't have had the tenacity to stick with this for the long haul without your years of guidance and encouragement.

To Marlys Barker, you gave a young newspaper reporter a chance all those years ago, and while working for you, I honed many of the skills necessary to write this book.

To Deanna, Chris, Marti, Wendy, Marisa, Cinnamon, Mara, and Rachel, thank you for walking alongside me after my diagnosis. You knew when to cry with me, when to laugh with me, and when to bring me coffee and doughnuts. Your friendship through cancer and your critiques of my early chapter drafts were invaluable.

To Dr. Susan Beck, thank you for responding to my cold call to your office, meeting me for coffee, and then proceeding to read through every chapter of my first draft to provide vital feedback and insight. I prayed for a year that God would provide a medical professional to come alongside me, and you were the answer.

To the women and men in this book who willingly relived extremely hard things as you shared your mastectomy and breast reconstruction experiences with me, thank you. We are connected in a way that we never would have chosen, but I am beyond grateful that your stories are now a part of my story.

To my Lord and Savior, Jesus, you had a purpose and plan for this cancer road and were a comforting presence every step of the way.

Foreword

I was doing rounds on my day's surgical patients when I received a call from Kim. She introduced herself and said a friend had recommended she call me. She was writing a book about her experience with mastectomy and breast reconstruction after a breast cancer diagnosis and wanted a female surgeon's perspective. I am a breast surgeon and medical director of a busy comprehensive breast center in Clive, Iowa. I was not Kim's surgeon, but we met in a coffee shop and exchanged stories of our encounters with breast cancer—hers so very personal and mine as a caregiver. She asked me to read her book, *Life Reconstructed*.

I received the first five chapters and read them carefully. My comprehension from a surgeon's perspective quickly shifted to the patient's point of view. I see women with breast cancer almost daily, and oftentimes I am the first person to give them the diagnosis, prognosis, and appropriate treatment recommendations. It is a mind-blowing amount of information, let alone the diagnosis itself. Kim's book took me beyond the office visit, operating room, and hospital experiences; she shares her heartbreak with her family and friends at home, before and after surgery. I learned so much from her experience and the experiences of women she interviewed from diagnosis to a cancer-free recovery. I was comforted by some of the experiences and humbled and disheartened by others.

Kim's journalistic skills and storytelling ability to share her own personal struggles with breast cancer make this book exceptional. She includes helpful insights on how to deal with the collateral damage perpetrated on family and friends after the diagnosis of breast cancer along with how her faith lifted her and her husband up daily. Their faith encouraged them to persevere through all the hardships and grief of this diagnosis.

It truly was a gift that Kim contacted me and asked me to read her story about her encounter with a disease that touches too many women, family, and friends. I have taken to heart all that she has shared in this book, and I think about her words every time I see another woman with breast cancer. Kim's story has made me a better and more holistic breast surgeon, and I now choose my multidisciplinary physician team to better match the physical and emotional needs of my patients.

Life Reconstructed is a must-read for anyone diagnosed with breast cancer and facing mastectomy and breast reconstruction, as well as for the spouses and friends sharing the cancer journey. I also challenge my surgical colleagues to read this story of one woman's experience with this diagnosis to fully understand the patient perspective.

Susan L. Beck, DO, MPH,

Breast Surgeon and Medical Director,

Katzmann Breast Center

Introduction

The World Turned Upside Down: When Breast Cancer Came to My House

This is not a cancer book. But because it was cancer that led to these words in print, it seems fitting that I invite you into my living room to observe the hardest night of my life: the night my husband and I told our three children about my diagnosis.

We sat in front of the fireplace, Corey and me. It was January 21, 2016—two days after my biopsy. Carter leaned against the living room wall, Owen against a couch, and Lewis beside him (our two teenagers and the nine-year-old who will always be my baby). A surreal, fear-tinged atmosphere surrounded that moment.

The boys knew about my biopsy. They knew something was not quite right with my body. But they were as ill-prepared for the blow as I was.

Invasive ductal carcinoma. Breast cancer. Corey and I had allowed ourselves twenty-four hours to process the news, and now it was time to bring the boys into this undesirable circle.

I couldn't physically voice my diagnosis to the boys. As I watched them quietly brace for whatever news was coming, the pathway from my vocal cords to my lips grew tight and suddenly there was not enough air in the room to form words. So I just leaned on Corey, hoping that somehow his strength would seep into me and praying that his words would not get lost like mine.

"We got the biopsy results back, and your mom has breast cancer." Silence.

The world stopped for a minute while we watched our boys' insulated lives burst wide open. Tears don't often flow freely at our house, but that night they did. I saw the fear in my boys' eyes, and more than anything, I wanted to take it away. *It's going to be okay. Breast cancer is treatable. The doctors will fix this, and then we'll get right back to normal* is what I wanted to say. But the truth is I was drowning in fear myself.

It was fear of the unknown—all I had at that point was a name for my tumor. I didn't know if it had spread beyond the lump I could feel under the skin of my breast. I didn't know what my future looked like. Chemo? Radiation? Surgery? Death? I just knew that something was growing inside of me that was not supposed to be and that I was helpless to stop it.

Overcoming Fear

Fear can do crazy things to your mind if you let it. It can take you down paths you don't want to be on. And I had days when all of my energy was spent fighting the ugly thought that I was full of cancer and going to die. But even as those thoughts bombarded me, one Bible verse kept coming to the forefront of my mind: "Do not fear, for I am with you; do not be dismayed, for I am your God. I will strengthen you and help you; I will uphold you with my righteous right hand." It's from the forty-first chapter of Isaiah, and I had memorized it during high school to get me through the jitters I always felt before the starting gun went off at a track meet. I couldn't have known at that time how much more I would need those words at age forty than I did at fifteen.

God may not play a role in your journey, but He is integral in mine.

The purpose of this book is not to convince you God is real, but my story would be only half-told if I did not include the role that faith played in my experience.

I'm unsure if I fully believed all the words of the Isaiah verse at that time, but the more I took the fear and covered it with "fear not," the more I trusted that God knew what He was doing. This book is interspersed with examples of how that worked in my life, that He wasn't looking down from heaven saying, "Oh shoot, I screwed that one up. Kim wasn't supposed to get that tumor. Oh well, she's got it now; I guess we'll go with it." I think what He wanted was for me to learn to trust Him in the hard stuff.

The Path through Treatment

The boys survived that night in the living room. They worked their way through the fear, and they helped me make it through a really tough season.

While recovering from my bilateral mastectomy and the first phase of reconstruction, a surgery that took nearly five hours, they (along with Corey) were my physical strength. They helped me out of the recliner. They opened the refrigerator door. They refilled my water bottle. They adjusted my footstool.

And they graciously kept being themselves as well. They still yelled at the Xbox when their games weren't going right, they still ate their way through a million boxes of cereal, they still wrestled on the living room floor, and they still got passionately involved in viewing Iowa State Cyclone basketball games on TV. Together, we found a new normal, and we grew to have a deep appreciation of each other and our time together.

While the boys helped me out and worked through those challenging months in their own way, Corey did hard things too. He came home at lunchtime to help me shower, he blew my hair dry and helped me get dressed, he emptied the surgical drains placed in my body to remove excess fluid in the first weeks of recovery, and he told me I was beautiful when my scars told me I was not.

Throughout my reconstruction process, which lasted about five months, he drove me to the plastic surgeon's office so many times I'm sure he could do it blindfolded. He watched Netflix with me late into the night when I couldn't get comfortable enough to sleep, and he convinced me that it was okay to call my doctor and request sleeping pills—a move that I'm convinced saved my sanity during those long, uncomfortable months.

On the Other Side

I am on the other side of cancer and reconstruction now. The cancer was scary. The reconstruction process was uncomfortable on good days and excruciating on bad days. But I persevered.

I can look back and see clearly that even in a disease like breast cancer, with its ugly physical scars that remain long after reconstruction is complete, beauty can be found. I have grown in ways that would not be possible without that unexpected bump in my road.

In the following pages, I want to share what I have learned with you. If you are going through breast reconstruction, your road will no doubt look different from mine, but our shared experience of mastectomy and reconstruction creates a bond between us, even if we never meet beyond the pages of this book.

In this book, I walk through my experience of dealing with and persevering through the physical and emotional toll that breast recon-struction took on me, and I share input from many women who have successfully navigated the challenges, both to mind and to body. I also include stories of living with reconstructed breasts, and how living post-reconstruction differs significantly from living post-augmentation (also known as a boob job). A glossary is also included, providing a non-exhaustive medical knowledge base of procedures and materials in layman's terms, as well as appendixes that list helpful items for recovery and information about the history of breast reconstruction and the laws in place to help you during this difficult journey.

Those going through this with a significant other know that the ordeal deeply affects the one who loves you most. In coming pages, I look at the process from a husband's perspective, having spoken with men who've walked the road with their wives. This season of life is hard on us women going through it, but it takes a toll on our men as well. If you are that someone who is on the breast reconstruction road with your partner, may these pages give you knowledge and understanding with which to care for and support your loved one.

Children are also affected deeply and are often fearful. One chapter looks at ways to involve children in the process at an age-appropriate level. Some kids are so young when cancer hits that all they know about this trial in their family is through stories they hear long after the fact. Other kids, like mine, were old enough to understand and needed to be kept in the loop for their emotional well-being.

Sex is a chapter topic as well. Corey and I had just celebrated our seventeenth wedding anniversary when I was diagnosed, and we thought we had the sex thing all figured out. My diagnosis and treatment rocked our world in the intimacy department. It has been challenging, and sex will never be the same as before, but it keeps improving. I am even confident that eventually it will be better than it ever was.

With my personal story, contributions from many women with various forms of breast reconstruction, input from the men who have supported them through it, and insights from medical professionals working in the reconstruction field, the following pages are informative, encouraging, and raw.

Hopefully you will hear my written words as a reassuring voice. Cancer is the hardest thing our family has ever done together, and the reconstruction process is a bizarre world to navigate. The circumstances of 2016 were most definitely not something I would have chosen, but in ways I've struggled putting words to, it was a beautiful experience.

Perhaps the most meaningful part is that I am alive to write this book—the book I wanted to read as I traveled down the reconstruction road. I hope that as you read the following words, you will feel as if I am a friend on the road by your side.

Chapter 1

Open to the Front: The Humbling Experience of Sharing Your Breasts with So Many People

"Beautiful girl, you can do hard things."
—Unknown

"Put this on, please. And make sure it's *open to the front*."

I quickly lost count of the number of times I heard that phrase coming from the mouth of a person wearing scrubs and holding out a pink paper vest.

There was something otherworldly about repeatedly slipping into a crinkly pink vest, knowing a few short minutes later I'd have to take it back off so a stranger in a white lab coat could get up close and personal with my boobs. Add to that awkwardness my brain struggling to wrap itself around the fact that I had cancer, and it was like I'd stepped out of normal life and into some sort of demented alternate reality.

On one hand, I totally wanted all the smart medical people to look at my boobs and squeeze them and push on them and photograph them and do all the things they needed to do to get me on my way to complete healing. On the other hand, I wanted to grab my magic blanket (my BFF gave me a sherpa blanket after my diagnosis), curl up in a ball on the floor in front of my fireplace, and just sleep until the whole thing was over.

When It Feels Like Your Boobs Are Public Property

It started with Dr. Testroet. She's our family doctor, she's my age, and I kind of feel like she's my friend. I've even considered pretending I was sick so I could sneak a couple coffees into the exam room and sit and chat with her about books and backpacking. But show her my boobs? Nah. That thought never crossed my mind.

Then on a cold and windy day in January 2016, I found a weird lump in my left breast and thought, *Oh crap. I should probably have that looked at.* So off to Dr. Testroet I went. I really wasn't worried at that point. I was only forty years old and had no breast cancer in my family history. A little voice in my head kept telling me I was being silly for even making the appointment and wasting the hard-earned money in our health savings account. Certainly it was nothing to be concerned about. I never imagined that I would soon hear those awful words, "You have breast cancer," and that Dr. Testroet would be the first of many people in the medical field to view and feel my breasts that year.

The mammogram lady was breast-toucher number two. Then it was the ultrasound lady, followed by the radiologist who did the biopsy. Then on to the general surgeon. Then plastic surgeon number one. (He is one I would rather forget. You will learn more about him in Chapter 4.) Then on to plastic surgeon number two. Then it was the oncologist and his assistant. Sprinkled into that mix were lots of nurses and three doctors in training:

"Do you mind if so-and-so sits in on this appointment? He's working on his residency . . ."

"That's fine" was my verbal answer, but internally the words were considerably more sarcastic—*Why, of course not. I want to show my boobs to as many people as possible before they are removed from my body and sent into the great unknown.*

The whole experience was super weird for me. Please know that if it's super weird for you too, you are not alone.

Thoughts from Women Who Have Been There

When Rachel was in her early teens, her mom was diagnosed with breast cancer. After treatment she lived cancer-free for several years, but it eventually came back and took her life when Rachel was in college, so Rachel knew from an early age that she would have to keep a close watch on her own breast health. But even with that knowledge, repeatedly revealing her boobs was really strange at first.

"The pictures [they took of my boobs] were really weird, but I remember the doctor talking about it afterward and [learning] that my pictures were going to end up in a reference book for other women in the same position as me. . . . Instead of being really weirded out by that, I thought about how thankful I was to have had the opportunity to flip through pages of before-and-after photos. When I thought about it that way, I didn't mind so much," she said. "Plus, my doctors worked hard to make it feel like it was okay, and that it was just another body part. I got used to it over time." (Many plastic surgeons take before-and-after photographs from the neck down and keep an album for new patients to view prior to their surgeries.)

Amber quickly became desensitized to exposing her boobs. At the beginning, she kept track of the number of people who looked at her breasts, but as that amount grew and grew through chemotherapy, radiation, and surgeries, she stopped counting. "Showing my breasts became normal; it lost the feel of being an intimate, private, sexual experience and became clinical," she said. "I still feel that way. Maybe because they are man-made!"

Krystal can relate to the clinical feeling. In fact, after going through the mastectomy and breast reconstruction process, she now feels comfortable showing her new breasts to other women to educate them about the process. "I've accepted that these are my new boobs, and when I explain what I've had done, sometimes it's easier to just show them," she said.

Cathy remembers the awkwardness of the first time she bared her breasts in her cancer journey. It was with her radiologist. He attended the same large church where Cathy led the drama ministry. He knew her because of her presence in ministry, but she didn't recognize him. So he casually chatted with her about their church connection and then abruptly switched from small talk to "Let's take a look at your breasts." Cathy had a hard time with the transition. "It just seemed so surreal. Such an easy transition for him and downright shocking to me."

She gradually grew used to the *open to the front* routine, but as her treatment was wrapping up, her reconstructive surgeon threw her for a loop. As he examined her healed breasts at a follow-up appointment after surgery, he stood back to admire his handiwork and said, "That's one of the best reconstructions I've ever seen."

We can't control what doctors, nurses, and other medical professionals say and do as they examine this intimate part of our bodies, but we can control how we handle the situation. Like everything in life, this whole out-of-this-world scenario will be easier for some people to deal with than others. If it's not uncomfortable for you, that's fantastic! One less thing to stress over throughout treatment. You might just want to skim through the rest of this chapter and move on to other topics. But if you are finding it difficult to make your way through these *open to the front* appointments, read on for some thoughts on coping.

Ideas for Coping with Repeated Boob Exposure

Regardless of where you land on the comfort-level spectrum, being thrown into a world where you have no choice but to repeatedly reveal your breasts while processing the fact that you have cancer is not a cakewalk. So don't try to pretend it is. Go ahead and settle in to that hard place. Cry all the tears. Get good and angry. Cover your face with a pillow and scream. Buy a punching bag and smack it around. Whatever you need to do to release the tension, the discomfort, and the fear, do that thing. And when you head into that exam room where it is inappropriate to scream and punch things, consider trying one of the following coping mechanisms:

- **Think of your situation as a challenge** rather than a threat. According to wellness coach and stress management specialist Elizabeth Scott, "Research shows that viewing something as a challenge helps you to mobilize your resources and bring your 'A game' to the situation more easily, while viewing the same situation as a threat can lead to a greater tendency to feel stressed and shut down."[1]

- **Focus on breathing.** Deep abdominal breathing has actual physical benefits. According to an article published by Harvard Medical School, deep abdominal breathing encourages full oxygen exchange, and doing so can slow the heartbeat and stabilize or even lower blood pressure.[2] (See sidebar for breathing techniques.)

- **Try mantra meditation.** Find a comforting scripture passage or motivational phrase to memorize, and meditate on those words as you endure the discomfort. According to the Mayo Clinic staff, meditation is a form of mind-body complementary medicine and it can produce relaxation and tranquility.[3] (See sidebar for suggestions.)

- **Try visual meditation.** The goal for visual meditation is to form mental images of places you find relaxing.[4] So let your mind leave the room during those breast exams; close your eyes and pretend you are in the mountains or on the beach, or wherever your happy place happens to be.

- **Chew gum.** According to a study published in the journal *Clinical Practice & Epidemiology in Mental Health*, two weeks of chewing gum twice per day lowered the anxiety levels of the test group.[5] So go ahead and grab some Trident on the way to your appointment.

Breathing Techniques

According to the American Institute of Stress (AIS), focused breathing is mentally active and leaves the body relaxed, calm, and focused.[6] Practicing breathing techniques helps you feel connected to your body. It takes your focus away from your worries and allows you to calm your mind.

Below is a brief overview of various breathing techniques (detailed at AIS and Anxieties.com) that can easily be practiced anywhere, including that little examination room where you so often sit with your pink vest *open to the front.*

- **Abdominal or Natural Breathing.** Gently inhale a normal amount of air through your nose, filling your lower lungs. Breathe out normally. Continue this pattern, focusing on filling the lower lungs. This technique provides sufficient oxygen and controls the exhalation of carbon dioxide.
- **Calming Breath.** Calming breath is a powerful way to control hyperventilation, slow a rapid heartbeat, and promote physical comfort.[7] To perform calming breath, take a long, slow breath through your nose, filling the lower lungs first and then the upper lungs. Hold your breath for a count of three. Then slowly exhale through pursed lips while relaxing the muscles

in your face, jaw, shoulders, and stomach. This should take about thirty seconds to complete.

- **Calming Counts.** Take a long, slow breath in and then exhale it while saying the word "relax" silently. Then close your eyes and take ten natural breaths, counting down from ten to one. While taking the ten natural breaths, keep your eyes closed and imagine your tensions loosening. When you reach "one," open your eyes. This technique should take about ninety seconds.

- **The Quieting Response.** The first step is to "smile inwardly with your eyes and mouth and release the tension in your shoulders."[8] (I don't know about you, but I carry most of my stress in my shoulders and neck, so this makes a lot of sense to me.) The next step is to imagine holes in the soles of your feet and breathe in. While breathing, visualize hot air entering your body through those holes and moving slowly up to your lungs. As the "hot air" moves up through your body, relax your muscles sequentially. Then, while exhaling, reverse the visualization so the hot air leaves your body through your feet. This technique can be performed in as little as six seconds.

Meditation

Consider memorizing one or more of the following inspirational quotes or scripture passages to repeat in your head as you endure the hard parts of your doctor appointments.

- "Therefore I tell you, do not worry about your life, what you will eat or drink; or about your body, what you will wear. Is not life more than food, and the body more than clothes? Look at the birds of the air; they do not sow or reap or store away in barns, and yet your heavenly Father feeds them. Are you not much more valuable than they? Can any one of you by worrying add a single hour to your life?" —Matthew 6:25–27 (NIV)

- "Trust yourself. You've survived a lot, and you'll survive whatever is happening right now, too." —Karen Salmansohn[9]
- "Even though I walk through the darkest valley, I will fear no evil, for you are with me; your rod and your staff, they comfort me." —Psalm 23:4 (NIV)
- "You can't control what goes on outside. But you can always control what goes on inside." —Wayne Dyer
- "Anxiety does not empty tomorrow of its sorrows, but only empties today of its strength." —Charles Spurgeon[10]
- "For I am the Lord your God who takes hold of your right hand and says to you, Do not fear; I will help you." —Isaiah 41:13 (NIV)
- "Life is ten percent what happens to me and ninety percent how I react to it." —Charles Swindoll
- "Come to me, all you who are weary and burdened, and I will give you rest. Take my yoke upon you and learn from me, for I am gentle and humble in heart, and you will find rest for your souls. For my yoke is easy and my burden is light." —Matthew 11:28–30 (NIV)
- "So do not fear, for I am with you; do not be dismayed, for I am your God. I will strengthen you and help you; I will uphold you with my righteous right hand." — Isaiah 41:10 (NIV)
- "Don't let your mind bully your body into believing

> it must carry the burden of its worries." —Terri Guillemets
>
> - "Do not fear, for I have redeemed you; I have summoned you by name; you are mine. When you pass through the waters, I will be with you; and when you pass through the rivers, they will not sweep over you. When you walk through the fire, you will not be burned; the flames will not set you ablaze. For I am the Lord your God, the Holy One of Israel, your Savior." —Isaiah 43:1–3 (NIV)
> - "We must be willing to let go of the life we have planned, so as to have the life that is waiting for us." —Joseph Campbell[11]
> - "You don't have to see the whole staircase. Just take the first step." —Martin Luther King Jr.

While these coping mechanisms can be helpful, you can try a variety of other techniques not listed here. Focus on what you *can* do, and try to be creative if none of these methods work for you. A few other ideas include: the following pinpoint a spot on the wall and focus on that spot while your shirt is off, count backward from one hundred down to one, or look for humor in the situation.

Humor was my savior. I did plenty of crying, and a little screaming as well (later, in the car or at home, after the exam was complete), but ultimately, humor became a key coping mechanism for me. Corey and I came up with a game called Tally the People Who Check Out My Boobs. We started keeping track of the number of people who looked at my breasts, and each time one of those blasted "doctors in residence" entered the room, I let myself be annoyed for a minute and then gave myself bonus points.

Maybe humor won't work for you, and that's okay. But I urge you to find a way that helps you get through those appointments with less tension and stress. The important thing is not the type of stress reliever you use but that you do something to ease the yucky feelings that can be overwhelming when your shirt comes off.

Looking Back

So many things about breast cancer are so awfully hard, not the least of which is sitting topless in front of relative strangers. But you can make it through this hard thing. It's like a lot of other hard things in life. You can't go around it, and you can't skip over it. You just have to make it step by painful step to the other side. And as time passes, it does get easier.

I have the benefit of hindsight. It's been a few years since I walked that crummy cancer road and all that goes with it. And when I think back to all the discomfort and awkwardness that came from people examining and touching my boobs, it feels like a blip on the radar of my life as a whole. A painful but necessary blip. A blip that was part of the process of healing my body, increasing my faith in God, giving me a new perspective on life, and giving me more time on this earth with my family.

Because of that, every poke, prod, and photograph was worth it.

Resources

1. Scott, Elizabeth. "How to Adapt to a Stressful Situation." *Verywell Mind*, reviewed November 10, 2019. https://www.verywellmind.com/how-to-adapt-to-a-stressful-situation-3144674.

2. Harvard Medical School. "Relaxation Techniques: Breath Control Helps Quell Errant Stress Response." Harvard Health Publishing, updated July 6, 2020. https://www.health.harvard.edu/mind-and-mood/relaxation-techniques-breath-control-helps-quell-errant-stress-response.

3. Mayo Clinic Staff. "Meditation: A Simple, Fast Way to Reduce Stress." MayoClinic.com, April 22, 2020. https://www.mayoclinic.org/tests-procedures/meditation/in-depth/meditation/art-20045858.

4. Ibid.

5. Sasaki-Otomaru, Akiyo; Sakuma, Yumiko; Mochizuki, Yoshiko; Ishida, Sadayo; Kanoya, Yuka; and Sato, Chifumi. 2011. "Effect of Regular Gum Chewing on Levels of Anxiety, Mood, and Fatigue in Healthy Young Adults." *Clinical Practice & Epidemiology in Mental Health* 7: 133–39. https://www.ncbi.nlm.nih.gov/pmc/articles/PMC3158435/.

6. Marksberry, Kellie. "Take a Deep Breath." The American Institute of Stress, August 10, 2012. https://www.stress.org/take-a-deep-breath/.

7. "Step 3: Breathe!" Anxieties.com, accessed December 2, 2019. https://www.anxieties.com/88/flying-step3#.xx_BgihKjD4.

8. Kellie Marksberry, "Take a Deep Breath."

9. Salmansohn, Karen. "25 Feeling Unloved Quotes for When You Don't Feel Loved." NotSalmon.com, accessed April 23, 2020. https://www.notsalmon.com/2015/08/14/quotes-about-unlove/.

10. Spurgeon, Charles. *The Salt-Cellars*. London: Passmore and Alabaster, 1889.

11. Osbon, Diane K. *Reflections on the Art of Living: A Joseph Campbell Companion*. New York: Harper Perennial, reprint edition, May 1, 1995.

Chapter 2

Breast Reconstruction: To Do It or Not to Do It

"I do not feel any less of a woman. I feel empowered
that I made a strong choice
that in no way diminishes my femininity."
—Angelina Jolie[1]

I think I was in fifth grade when I asked my mom for a training bra. I wasn't sure exactly how a bra was going to train my boobs, but I did know that I was the only one of my friends without one. And when you are eleven, being the girl without the bra is torture. It took me weeks to work up the nerve to ask for this intimate item of clothing, but after I did, I came home from school to find training bras on my bed.

I happily wore those bras until I graduated to a real one. But to be honest, aside from the nipple factor, I never really needed a bra. I'm a petite, 5-foot-3-inch-tall woman, and the only time my boobs were big enough to necessitate support was when I was pregnant and nursing babies. In fact, prior to my **bilateral (double) mastectomy** (a surgery to remove all the tissue of both breasts), I bought all my bras in the girls' section at Kohl's. And no, I'm not talking about the juniors' section; I'm talking about the little girls' I'm-progressing-from-a-training-bra-to-a-real-bra section.

My chest size didn't concern me much. It's just the way things were. Filling out even the smallest of women's bra cups was an impossible dream, and I was okay with that for the most part. I know I could have stuffed a woman's bra or worn a padded one, but that just wasn't me. Plus, as it turns out, the bras in the girls' section are half the price of adult bras. A happy consequence of having a small chest.

My Ugly Boobs

Though my small chest never really bothered me, by the time I was diagnosed with cancer, I didn't like my breasts. After breastfeeding, they lost the little volume they had, and they were ugly to me. It's like my boobs disappeared, and in their place were droopy nipples attached to saggy boob skin. But even so, I couldn't envision myself without breasts. In fact, I actually had the thought, *Well, this cancer thing sucks, but maybe at the end of it I won't have prepubescent-sized boobs with geriatric-like sags.*

A part of me looked forward to having boobs that wouldn't leave gaping empty spaces in bra cups. It was for that reason, and for the sake of my husband, that I didn't consider **going flat** (opting not to go through reconstruction after a mastectomy, which is a perfectly acceptable choice).

I can confidently say I know that Corey would have supported me fully if I had chosen to go flat, but I've been married to him for eighteen years and I know my looks affect him sexually. And I don't mean that he only loves me for my body, but that God created him to see beauty in my breasts, and (unlike me) he actually thoroughly enjoyed my small, saggy old-lady boobs. So I wanted to love my husband by having my breasts reconstructed.

But not every woman feels the same as me. And not every husband is built like mine. And that's okay. There is no right or wrong answer to the question of breast reconstruction versus going flat. It's an intensely personal choice, and women opt for and against reconstruction for a variety of reasons. We'd all choose healthy, cancer-free natural breasts if we could. Unfortunately for us, that choice is off the table.

In this chapter, I will take you briefly into the journeys of a number of women who faced this choice. Women who, either because of a cancer diagnosis or a genetic mutation for the disease, had to make a decision regarding the future of their breasts. Hopefully through their stories, you will gain some insight into which choice works the best for you or receive affirmation for the choice you already made.

Going Flat

Jodi

Jodi was forty-six years old when she was diagnosed with breast cancer. For the third year in a row, she was called back after her annual mammogram for a closer look. This time she was sent straight to ultrasound, which led to a biopsy, which was the beginning of her cancer road. That road included sixteen rounds of chemo, a bilateral mastectomy, and radiation.

She knew from the start that she would not have her breasts reconstructed. She was so confident of what she wanted that when her doctor suggested she talk to a plastic surgeon before making the decision, she refused.

"I knew without a doubt I didn't want it. I didn't want anything else put in my body. I was getting stuff out that wasn't supposed to be there, and I didn't want to put anything else in there. I guess I just felt that my breasts didn't define who I was, so I was okay with not having them."

Though I chose a different road than Jodi, she speaks truth. Our culture tries to lead us to believe that our value lies in our breasts, our weight, and our wrinkle-free skin, but our culture speaks lies. We are not greater or lesser as women because of our breasts. Our value lies in our spirit, not our cup size.

Vickie

Vickie also decided to go flat. Diagnosed with breast cancer at age sixty-four, she underwent radiation, four rounds of chemo, and a **unilateral (single) mastectomy** (a surgery to remove the tissue of a single breast*). Several factors played a role in Vickie's decision. Age** and the physical toll of another surgery worked into her decision-making process, but they were secondary to her firm belief that she wouldn't miss her breasts.

"I thought I'd really miss an arm or a leg or an eye, but a breast? A breast doesn't really function after you are done nursing your babies, except to make clothes fit, and you can do that with a **prosthesis**" (a breast mold made to mimic a natural breast that can be placed in the bra when desired).

The hardest part of making the decision for Vickie was that everyone she discussed it with thought she should have reconstruction. Her husband, Steve, feared she would later regret the decision, but after listening to her arguments, he realized she was certain.

"Until I really thought about who my wife was, I was afraid that some time down the road she'd regret her decision. But she's not like that. She's the type of person who knows what she wants. And when she makes a decision, she sticks with it," he said.

Years later, she is still content with her flat chest and comfortable with her prosthesis.

---

* Approximately 99 percent of breast tissue is removed during a mastectomy. Because of the makeup of the breast, it is impossible to be assured that 100 percent of the tissue is removed.

** Older patients assume that they are at a higher risk of complications than younger women. However, a recent study in the *Journal of the American College of Surgeons* found that age holds little weight when it comes to complications following reconstruction surgery. In more than 1500 women observed, those under age forty-five and those over sixty had similar complication rates.[2]

Sara Bartosiewicz-Hamilton

Sara Bartosiewicz-Hamilton is a breast cancer **previvor** (a woman who undergoes a bilateral mastectomy prior to a cancer diagnosis). Mastectomies are not only performed on breast cancer patients but are also a treatment option for women who are cancer-free and have tested positive for the gene mutation for the disease on their BRCA1 or BRCA2 gene. This mutation greatly increases their breast cancer risk for the future.

After testing positive for the BRCA2 gene mutation in 2006, Sara had a **prophylactic bilateral mastectomy** (a mastectomy performed prior to a cancer diagnosis) and went through the reconstruction process. Resulting complications from two different types of implants, however, led her to later have them removed and go flat.

Sara, who founded the online support group Flatandfabulous.org, believes it's common for women to feel judged when they don't choose reconstruction. "It's wrapped up in what society believes a woman should look like and that my identity is wrapped up in two breasts, whether they are mine or not."

Sara considers herself very feminine, and one of her missions through Flat & Fabulous is to focus on empowerment. "People should live life to the fullest without worrying what society or their moms or best friends think, because at the end of the day you're going to look back on your life and need to make it the best life you can possibly live."[3]

More Women Are Going Flat

It's common for women who choose to go flat to feel like they are a part of a small minority, but they're not. Though there are conflicting numbers from different studies, according to Breastcancer.org, a 2014 study showed that 44 percent of women who underwent mastectomies didn't undergo reconstruction.[4] Flatandfabulous.org claims that percentage is even higher.

Breast surgeon Dr. Deanna J. Attai, a past president of the American Society of Breast Surgeons, said the number of her patients opting out of reconstruction is growing. "Sometimes women feel like it's just too much: It's too involved, there are too many steps, it's too long a process," she told the *New York Times*.[5]

Going flat is the best decision for many women, and there is a growing network of support for women who choose this route. And for women who choose to go flat but don't necessarily want to look flat, prostheses are an option.

Prostheses

Both Jodi and Vickie chose to use prostheses. Prostheses are covered by insurance through the Women's Health and Cancer Rights Act (see Appendix 2), and each woman is fitted for prostheses specific to her body. This requires a trip to a Certified Breast Prosthesis Fitter to be measured to determine the cup size that will look most natural and, if the woman is getting a single prosthesis, the size and shape that will best match the remaining breast. They are most commonly made of silicone (but foam or fiberfill covered in a fabric like cotton) encased in a plastic sheath.

Vickie wears her silicone prosthesis every day and said it wasn't hard getting used to, though in the hot summer sun she opts for a lighter-weight cotton one. Breast prostheses give women without a breast a natural look in their clothing. Plunging necklines and swimwear can still pose a challenge, but the majority of women who have undergone mastectomies can wear most anything without giving away that they are missing one or both breasts.

Some Thoughts on Going Flat from a Breast Surgeon

Breast surgeon Susan Beck, DO, began her career as a general and breast surgeon in 1989 but committed solely to breast surgery in 2006.

In that time, she's worked with a diverse number of women who have chosen a wide variety of solutions in regard to mastectomy and breast reconstruction. Though some women are ultimately happy with their flat results, she said many of them think it's going to be easier than reconstruction, but that is not always the case.

"I tell my patients it's okay if they go flat, but it's not necessarily easier. You may still need revisional surgery later due to excess tissue."[6]

Revisional surgery is done to remove **dog ears** (pockets of fat under the arms after mastectomy) as well as skin bulges at the end of the scar or underneath the incision. Women with reconstructed breasts generally don't have issues with dog ears because that tissue is pulled into the breast as part of the reconstruction process. The skin bulges on the scars are also less noticeable on reconstructed breasts than on those who choose to go flat.

Beck said another thing to consider when contemplating going flat is that you will be able to see your tummy, and that makes some women struggle with body image. "I don't care how thin you are, when you go flat you are going to see your tummy," she said. "And you may feel like you are bloated even if you are not. It's just that you see it now and you didn't before."

Although going flat is the best choice for some women, it is not necessarily the easier option. It just involves a different set of possible complications compared to the complications that can arise with reconstructive surgery.

Choosing Reconstruction

Cathy

Cathy was encouraged to have a unilateral mastectomy after being diagnosed with breast cancer at age forty. She immediately knew she would undergo reconstruction to match her remaining natural breast.

She said, "I remember having the thought, 'I am not going to stuff my bra for the rest of my life.'" Cathy's reconstruction took place in 2000, and two decades later she has no regrets and has seen God at work through the whole process. "Deciding on reconstruction wasn't a faith decision for me, but faith was huge in being at peace throughout all of it and in accepting outcomes."

Though she's had no complications with her reconstructed breast, several years ago she revisited her plastic surgeon to have her natural breast "tweaked." Cathy found herself frustrated because her clothes stopped fitting right, and it was impossible to find a bra that worked for her body. "I was so out of balance," she said. "It was a vanity surgery, but I didn't care. I did it and I felt much better afterwards. And still do."

Over time, it's common for the two breasts to become lopsided in women who had a unilateral mastectomy with reconstruction. When this occurs, surgery can bring uniformity back to the breasts. (This type of surgery is included as part of breast cancer treatment in the Women's Health and Cancer Rights Act.[7])

Tammy

Diagnosed at age thirty, Tammy couldn't imagine living the rest of her life without breasts. She was confident from the outset that she wanted to have them reconstructed. And her feelings were confirmed over time as she lived for several months post-mastectomy with a flat chest. Because of her intense cancer treatment regimen, she was forced to delay reconstruction for almost a year after her bilateral mastectomy. By the time she finished chemo and radiation, she just wanted to feel whole and normal again.

"I felt like [not having reconstruction] would have been a constant reminder that I was sick. And now, because it's been so long and this is just what I look like, I don't think about it anymore. This is just what my body looks like. Maybe I would have come to those terms too, if I didn't do [reconstruction], but I don't think so. I think that it would've felt to me like I was still a sick person."

It's been twenty years since her reconstruction and she lives a full, active life, which includes water sports and other outdoor adventures. She said there have been only a couple times that she wished she could utilize the back muscle that is now a part of her breast. Other muscles compensate though, and she has no regrets.

Rachel

Rachel was twenty years old when her mom died of breast cancer. At age thirty-five, because of the high rate of cancer in her family, Rachel tested for the genetic mutation for the disease. She, along with two of her three sisters, tested positive for the BRCA2 mutation. Rachel chose to have a prophylactic bilateral mastectomy with reconstruction. She said she was 95 percent sure from the beginning of the process that she wanted to have reconstruction.

"I couldn't wrap my head around not having boobs," she said. "Plus, I swim at the Y, and I didn't want to deal with funny looks and pointing fingers in the locker room. I just don't think I could emotionally handle that."

Rachel said the tougher question for her was whether or not to go through with the bilateral mastectomy since she didn't actually have cancer. The decision was a hard one to make—until she had a biopsy scare.

That scare made her decision for her. After finding a spot in her MRI, her doctor scheduled a biopsy. She waited two weeks for her biopsy appointment and then another two days for results. Though it came back negative, she never wanted to go through that again. "I'd just be waiting for it to be positive. Every time," she said. "I couldn't live with that stress every six months. It'd kill me."

Going Flat Now and Changing Your Mind Later

The decision to undergo breast reconstruction is one that can be revisited later in life. A woman can change her mind years after her mastectomy and insurance is still required to pay for it as part of their breast cancer treatment coverage.

Kerry

Kerry was diagnosed with breast cancer when she was thirty-nine years old. At the time, she had three daughters aged thirteen and younger who kept her on her toes. She chose to go flat after her single mastectomy in order to get back to normal life as quickly as possible.

"Initially it was all so traumatic. I think I just wanted to get past the whole thing and move on," she said.

For almost twenty years, Kerry remained flat on one side. She didn't mind the prosthesis at first, but she never felt comfortable wearing anything sleeveless, and swimming suits didn't work for her despite several attempts with various prostheses.

It was after Kerry lost some weight and decided that she wanted to be able to wear sleeveless shirts and go swimming that she started thinking about reconstruction. "In the back of my mind, for a long time I thought, 'If I ever get breast cancer again, I'm doing reconstruction.'"

When an abnormal mammogram on her remaining breast led to a second cancer diagnosis nearly twenty years after her first, she didn't hesitate to choose reconstruction. She underwent a second unilateral mastectomy with reconstruction on both sides and found herself comfortable in a swimsuit after two decades of avoiding the pool.

Kerry doesn't regret choosing to go flat even though she later changed her mind. She just considers it all a part of her journey and is confident God was with her at every turn. "I would say that throughout the whole process, my faith in God provided the confidence that He was for me in this, just as He was for me in everything else in my life."

Some Reconstruction Thoughts from a Breast Surgeon

When you choose the reconstruction route, the size of your completed breasts is something that needs to be considered. Susan Beck, DO, says size is ultimately the woman's choice, but it's best not to go considerably larger than the size of the natural breasts. "I always tell my patients to remember to match their breast size with their frame."[8] Women who choose extra-large implants that don't fit their body type tend to have issues with skin tightness. These implants also tend to be heavy and hard, which can lead to discomfort.

It's valuable to do your research on types of reconstructive surgery. Beck said from her experience, implants are far more popular than flap (DIEP, TRAM, or latissimus) reconstruction, but both can be successful. However, she cautions that flap reconstruction means a bigger surgery, which adds risk of bigger complications. "Sometimes one side will take and the other one won't, and the patient will have to have an implant on one side. And some women think that by using tissue from their tummy they will be getting a bonus tummy tuck, but that's really not the case."

Questions to Guide the Decision-Making Process

One thing I have learned after going through the reconstruction process and speaking to many women of different ages, backgrounds, and viewpoints who were forced down the same road as me is that the right choice in regard to reconstruction is as varied as the women faced with the decision. Your right choice and my right choice may look very different. But regardless of the different outcomes, it is an unfortunate choice that has to be made.

The following is a list of questions designed to help women who are in the throes of making this life-altering decision:

- Do you currently have a healthy self-image? Do you think you will struggle with your self-image if you go flat?

- Do you, like Cathy, hate the idea of "stuffing your bra" for the rest of your life, but don't want to be flat chested?
- Do you, like Tammy, think that a flat chest would always serve as a reminder of when you were sick?
- Can your body physically handle more surgery? Do you have any physical ailments that would make recovery more arduous? (Diabetes? Bleeding disorders?)
- Do you, like Rachel, spend a lot of time in the pool? Is it important for you to look normal in a swimsuit or in the locker room while changing?
- Have you hit the limit of what you can handle, medically speaking? Are you just ready to be done?
- Like Jodi, does the thought of having a foreign object permanently implanted in your body bother you?
- Are you okay with having breasts that look similar to natural breasts but don't operate like natural breasts?
- Will going flat affect how you think about yourself sexually?
- If you are married, do you value your husband's opinion in this arena? If so, ask him for his thoughts and be prepared to let them hold some weight in your decision-making process.
- If faith plays a role in your life, might prayer and meditation help you come to a decision?

Some women immediately know without a doubt whether they want to undergo breast reconstruction or go flat after a mastectomy. Others don't. It can be a difficult decision, and it's one that no one can make for you. Hopefully the stories and tips in this chapter will help you make the decision that's right for *you*.

Resources

1. Barkhorn, Eleanor. "Angelina Jolie Is Still a Woman." *The Atlantic*, May 14, 2013. https://www.theatlantic.com/sexes/archive/2013/05/angelina-jolie-is-still-a-woman/275835/.

2. Santosa, Katherine B.; Qi, Ji; Kim, Hyungjin M.; Hamill, Jennifer B.; Pusic, Andrea L.; and Wilkins, Edwin G. 2016. "Effect of Patient Age on Outcomes in Breast Reconstruction: Results from a Multicenter Prospective Study." *Journal of the American College of Surgeons* 223, no. 6: 745–54. http://www.journalacs.org/article/S1072-7515(16)31451-X/fulltext.

3. Shulman, Leigh. "The Most Perfect Advice for Breast Cancer Awareness." Cloudhead.org, October 24, 2013. http://cloudhead.org/2013/10/24/most-perfect-advice-breast-cancer-awareness/.

4. "Going Flat: Choosing No Reconstruction." Breastcancer.org, updated March 7, 2019. https://www.breastcancer.org/treatment/surgery/reconstruction/no-reconstruction.

5. Rabin, Roni Caryn. "'Going Flat' After Breast Cancer." *New York Times*, October 31, 2016. https://www.nytimes.com/2016/11/01/well/live/going-flat-after-breast-cancer.html?_r=0.

6. Beck, Susan, DO. Interview by author. Huxley, Iowa, September 28, 2019.

7. "Women's Health and Cancer Rights Act." American Cancer Society, updated May 13, 2019. https://www.cancer.org/treatment/finding-and-paying-for-treatment/understanding-health-insurance/health-insurance-laws/womens-health-and-cancer-rights-act.html.

8. Susan Beck, interview by author.

Chapter 3

It's Not a Boob Job: The Distinct Differences between Reconstruction and Augmentation

"The biggest similarity between a breast augmentation appointment and a breast reconstruction appointment is the same pink paper gown that women wear open to the front."
—Jess Ludwig, RN[1]

I have no feeling in my breasts. So when people refer to breast reconstruction as a **boob job (breast augmentation)**, I kind of want to throat-punch them. That probably sounds a little brash, but it's like a dagger to my heart when someone compares the surgery I was forced into because of cancer to a surgery that's purely cosmetic.

If "boob job" and "breast reconstruction" were truly interchangeable terms, I'm convinced boob jobs would not exist. Who would choose to increase their bust size with side effects like long scars running across the center of each breast, no nipples, and completely severed nerve endings? And the emotional side effects that come with the removal of all the natural breast tissue can be even harder to overcome than the physical. Breast reconstruction is life altering. And because cancer is most often what makes reconstruction necessary, it's also, more often than not, bathed in heartbreak. A boob job is not.

When I was newly diagnosed with breast cancer and began frequenting medical clinics, I knew nothing about breast reconstruction procedures, the intensity of the process, the expected results, or the side effects. And although I knew breast augmentation and breast reconstruction were different animals, I didn't understand just how different. I certainly didn't feel educated enough to explain to someone how what I was about to go through would be exponentially harder than the experience of their cousin who had a boob job last year.

The further I traveled down the reconstruction road, and the more I researched, the better I understood that these two things that seem similar at a glance are so very different. And I want to share my experience and arsenal of knowledge with you.

Breast Reconstruction vs. Breast Augmentation— What's the Difference?

The most obvious difference between these two types of surgery is the reason they are performed. Breast reconstruction is necessary to restore breasts after a mastectomy. A variety of types of mastectomies exist based on the specifics of the surgical procedures and how much tissue is removed. But regardless of the procedure, a **mastectomy** removes about 99 percent of the breast tissue.

After my bilateral mastectomy, my plastic surgeon was tasked with creating something out of nothing. Tears drip onto my keyboard as I think about pieces of my feminine body being literally cut off and dug out, but that is exactly what happened on the morning of February 25, 2016.

After my general surgeon spent two and a half hours taking me apart, my plastic surgeon came in and spent another two and a half hours putting me back together. He had to clean up the mess. But even after this surgery, I was left with four-inch-long angry-looking incisions. (A few years later, those incisions calmed themselves down to soft pink scars.) Though not every woman has the same type of mastectomy or the same type of reconstruction I did, the pain of having a piece of yourself forever taken from you is universal.

Many women, including myself, who undergo **implant reconstruction** (inserting an implant that's filled with saline or silicone gel) are required to make a lot of trips to their plastic surgeon for **expansion appointments** (the slow stretching of skin, and sometimes muscle, to accommodate an implant). The expansion process is made possible by filling an **tissue expander** (a hard balloon-like device) that is placed in the chest during the first phase of reconstruction. The plastic surgeon pumps saline into each newly created breast through a menacingly long needle attached to a syringe.

After my best expansion appointments, I was uncomfortable for a couple days. After my worst ones, the pain was so intense that I had to sleep all night upright in my chair. Even the smallest movement made me feel like my chest might explode. I know my plastic surgeon would have removed some of the saline for me if I'd asked. In fact, he often told me if it was too uncomfortable (he didn't like to use the word "pain"), he would take some out. Unfortunately, it was never until after I arrived home from my appointment that the extent of the pain I would be enduring became evident. The idea of moving my screaming chest back into a car and driving forty minutes to the surgeon's office did not appeal to me, and I couldn't bear the thought of taking a step backwards. I just wanted to get done. I wanted to have all of this behind me and feel normal again. The removal of saline meant adding at least another week to my expansion schedule and thus pushing "normal" further away.

Not everyone has expanders as a part of their reconstruction experience. **Direct-to-implant** reconstruction is becoming more common. In direct-to-implant, reconstruction is completed immediately following a mastectomy and the months-long expansion process is eliminated.

In other instances, women undergo **flap reconstruction**, which uses tissue transplanted from another part of the body, such as the belly, thigh, or back. This frees women from the pain of expansion appointments, but it adds an extra layer of depth to their recovery (as they have multiple surgical sites and a longer overall time in surgery). Regardless of the type of reconstruction, women going through the process can endure pain for weeks. Even months.

But it's not just the physical pain of reconstruction that makes it differ from a boob job. Reconstruction comes from a place of sadness and loss. It's an attempt to regain a sense of normalcy after one of the key feminine parts of the body is removed. To this day I don't feel like my old self. I've found a new normal, but my breasts are not a part of the original me, and they never will be. And that makes me sad.

Breast augmentation, on the other hand, is what I consider a "happy procedure." It's something women do to improve their look, not to save their lives. During a **breast augmentation**, the plastic surgeon utilizes implants or fat to enhance the size and shape of already-existing breasts. The woman's natural breast tissue remains intact, expansion appointments are not necessary, and an implant is added to the breast tissue for aesthetic reasons. A breast augmentation is completed using a small incision in an inconspicuous area like the armpit or the underside of the areola, or even near the belly button.[2]

Though it is generally recommended to wait several weeks after an augmentation before resuming physically demanding tasks, the acute pain tends to ease up after the first few days. It also usually only requires a couple appointments with a plastic surgeon—a consult prior to surgery and a checkup after.

The procedures for reconstruction and augmentation bear some similarities—the same types of implants are used in both breast augmentation and breast reconstruction—but breast reconstruction is exponentially more challenging, both physically and emotionally.

Day-to-Day Life with Reconstructed Breasts

Not only do the surgery and recovery time for breast reconstruction and breast augmentation differ, but so do the end results. Each woman who undergoes breast reconstruction has a unique recovery experience and a unique assortment of aftereffects, but I have yet to meet a woman who has called her journey through reconstruction "easy."

From dealing with breast firmness and numbness, to lack of nipples, to the adverse effects reconstructed breasts can have on a sex life—the challenges are extensive. Between the physical pain and the emotional strain, I have cried more tears in the few years since cancer than in the decade prior.

Your experience will be unique to you, but you will likely face some bumps in the road. I will list some difficulties or obstacles you may experience as well as compare these challenges with a boob job so you can better understand (and explain to others if necessary) the important differences.

Nipples

To keep them or not to keep them. That is the question. Oh, the choices a woman never imagines she will have to make.

I had my nipples removed. Because of where my tumor developed, the **margins** (a rim of normal tissue surrounding the cancerous tissue) the surgeon needed to take affected my nipple area. I didn't really have a choice, but I think I would have decided to remove them if I did. I just knew I wanted all of my breast tissue gone for my peace of mind.

I later got nipple tattoos that look remarkably nice, though it would be hard to mistake them for the real thing. In fact, Corey and I joke about having a six-foot rule. If he stands about six feet away and gives my breasts a quick glance, he is almost convinced that I have real nipples. It's not perfect, but it's our attempt at making the best of this crazy circumstance life threw at us.

I had my tattooing done by Jenny,* an **aestheticist** (a medical tattoo artist) at a plastic surgeon's clinic. It was a surreal experience. I reclined topless in what kind of looked like a dentist chair while Corey sat in a chair near the door. The three of us talked about parenting and tropical vacations while Harry Connick Jr. Christmas music pumped through the speakers and ink pumped through Jenny's needle into my breasts. Bizarro.

Jenny used different ink tones and shading around the center of the tattoos to create a three-dimensional look on my two-dimensional nipples. A downside of medical tattoos is that they fade over time because the ink used for these tattoos is different from permanent commercial tattoo ink used in tattoo parlors. I'm told it's common for women who choose to go this route to have their tattoos touched up about every five years, but I didn't make it that long. Mine started fading out within a year, so I had a second visit with Jenny.

Some women who undergo nipple removal with their bilateral mastectomies choose to have an additional surgery to re-create nipples. During this outpatient surgery, the plastic surgeon makes a small incision, forms a nipple shape with the breast skin, and holds it in place with stitches until it heals. (In some instances, skin is grafted from the inner thigh or labia instead.) Though reconstructing the nipple provides a more natural-looking breast than tattooing alone, reconstructed nipples can flatten out or fall over time, requiring more surgery.

For other women, a **nipple-sparing mastectomy** is an option. This is dependent on a number of factors, including the type of

---

* Name changed for privacy.

cancer, the size of the tumor(s), and the tumor location within the breast. During a nipple-sparing mastectomy, the nipple is kept intact and allows the woman to retain a small portion of her natural breast. Though the nipple is natural, it's 100 percent aesthetic. The nerve endings are still severed, leaving the area void of sensation.

Misty, a thirty-something breast cancer survivor, chose to have a nipple-sparing mastectomy. "They do look different than before, but I'm happy with the outcome," she said. "No regrets. I've learned everything in this journey is a process to work through, and it takes time to adjust to the new you—physically, mentally, and emotionally."

A final nipple option is to have them removed and skip reconstruction and tattoos altogether. There is no right or wrong choice, and you can even wait years before deciding to go in for a nipple reconstruction surgery.

A Boob Job, in Comparison

Breast augmentation preserves natural nipples and usually preserves nipple sensation. But because the nerve that takes sensation to the nipple is thin and small, there is a risk of it getting cut or stretched during breast augmentation surgery. If it's stretched, the feeling generally comes back, but this can take up to two years. If it's cut, the damage is permanent. In the US, the risk of permanent nipple numbness after augmentation is 15 percent.[3]

Nerve Endings and Numbness

I have sensation around the perimeter of my breasts, but for the most part, my boobs feel the same way my cheeks feel after having a cavity filled. Annoyingly numb.

When Corey touches the tattoos where my nipples used to be, I have zero sensation. I've grown accustomed to it, but it still makes me sad sometimes. Especially when it comes to sexual intimacy. Like many women, I found my nipples to be one of the most sensitive parts of my body—a part that played a key role in sexual stimulation. I physically healed a long time ago, but Corey and I are still adjusting to this change in how my body responds to him. It's been a battle, and we've had more than one night of intimacy halted by tears. Sometimes mine. Sometimes his. But we are committed to working through the challenges because we long for the day that we can say we've overcome this obstacle.

During a mastectomy, the nerves of the breast are completely severed. Reconstruction made my breasts look nearly normal, but they don't feel normal. Some women experience regrowth of some nerve endings, but even with that regrowth, the sensation in the breast is different from before surgery.

A handful of years after previvor Rachel's bilateral mastectomy and reconstruction surgeries, very little feeling returned to her breasts. Numbness became the norm. She would take feeling back in a heartbeat if given the choice, but the lack of sensation doesn't disrupt her daily life.

"I'm constantly aware that it feels different, and there was a learning curve in getting used to it. But different is my normal now."

Though still rare, recent developments in breast reconstruction surgery have opened the door for some women to have breast sensation restored. It's not an option for women with implant reconstruction, but some plastic surgeons are now able to connect nerves in the flap tissue to nerves in the chest tissue during flap reconstruction surgery. The connected nerve fibers then regenerate and can gradually bring sensation back to the breasts.[4]

A Boob Job, in Comparison

Though women with breast augmentation may experience a change in the sensitivity of their breasts, the majority retain fully (or mostly) intact nerves. Some changes in sensation are likely felt as the body heals, but if the procedure is done right, the end result includes functioning nerve endings. This allows the woman to have enhanced breasts that feel the same sensations as her pre-surgery breasts.

According to a study published in *Plastic and Reconstructive Surgery*, the American Society of Plastic Surgeons' medical journal, 40 percent of women had some numbness after breast augmentation surgery, but only 2 percent had persistent numbness after healing.[5] One hundred percent of reconstruction patients deal with varying degrees of permanent numbness.

Breastfeeding

One of the most ridiculous things I read during the course of my breast cancer year was in a mastectomy informational booklet. It said, "It is unlikely that a woman will be able to breastfeed after a bilateral mastectomy."

Understatement, anyone? Corey and I had a good laugh after reading that.

A bilateral mastectomy removes all breast tissue. The milk ducts are gone. And the nipples from which milk exits the body are gone as well. Unlikely? How about utterly impossible?

My youngest was in second grade when I was diagnosed and we had no plans to add to our family, so this didn't affect me. But it's disappointing and even heartbreaking for a woman in her childbearing years to be stripped of her ability to breastfeed babies. Many women consider breastfeeding one of the most important experiences they share with their infants.

This rang painfully true for Tammy, a young mom of a toddler and a baby, when she was diagnosed with breast cancer. A couple years after successfully completing treatment, her third child was born. She found breastfeeding to be a special bonding experience with her first two babies, but it was not an option with her last. She said it was hard at first, but she kept things in perspective. She knew that having a third child was only possible because she made it through treatment alive and healthy. That trumped the disappointment.

She said, "When I look back at it, I don't feel that I missed anything [by not breastfeeding]. A breast cancer diagnosis makes you reevaluate what is important in life, and I was just very grateful to have a healthy baby."

A Boob Job, in Comparison

Most women who undergo breast augmentation are still able to breastfeed if they choose to do so. Though a small risk of damage occurring during surgery (that reduces a woman's ability to breastfeed) still exists, in most cases, all of the parts of the breast necessary for lactation remain functional.[6]

Scars

When I look at my naked torso in the mirror, I see pink four-inch scars running horizontally across each breast. They are a daily reminder of a very scary time in my life. Women who go the DIEP flap route (explained more in Chapter 4) have additional scarring from hip to hip on their abdomen. Like my breast scars, the abdominal scars fade over time, but they will never go away. Each scar forever serves as a reminder of what cancer took from us.

On the flip side, I think we can also look at our scars as a sign of strength—a reminder that we endured some really challenging stuff in order to stick around this earth for a while longer. Each morning when I look in the mirror, those scars encourage me to not take this life for granted.

Scars are weird like that, aren't they? They always represent something hard, because scars do not come without pain, but they can also represent healing and hope—a reminder of the suffering along with encouragement in the hope that healing brings.

A Boob Job, in Comparison

During a breast augmentation, a small incision is made in an inconspicuous area, resulting in little visible scarring. The incision is generally done around the areola, in the armpit, or on the underside of the breast. Sometimes it is even done at the navel, and the surgeon uses an endoscope to guide implant placement. After recovery, a woman who has undergone breast augmentation has a natural-looking and normal-feeling breast.

Firmness

I used to be a tummy sleeper. Not anymore. When I lie on my belly, it feels as if I have two tennis ball halves where my soft breast tissue should be. If you took a cross-section of my breasts, you would see the skin, layered on top of chest muscle, layered on top of a silicone implant, layered on top of the chest wall—no soft breast tissue.

Though I am getting used to the odd firmness of my breasts, I miss the softness of my real ones. To look at me clothed, you would never know that my breasts don't feel or function like real breasts, but every time I hug someone, my radar goes up and I wonder, *Can she feel that my breasts are weird? Because I can totally feel that my breasts are weird.*

Women who opt to use their own tissue for reconstruction have the benefit of more natural-feeling breasts than those who go the implant route. Judi originally had silicone implants but recently chose to have them removed and underwent DIEP flap surgery. Though her chest still remains numb, she loves the softness of her new breasts compared to the implants. "The feel of the breasts are very, very soft and squishy. They really are like *real* breasts. Droops and all!"

A Boob Job, in Comparison

Because women who undergo breast augmentation retain their breast tissue, they also retain the soft, natural feel of the breast. Breast augmentation has all the positives of breast reconstruction (if you can consider any part of breast reconstruction to be positive) and very few of the negatives.

Movement

Several years ago, our family watched the movie *Journey 2: The Mysterious Island*. A scene that my then elementary-age boys found particularly hilarious was when Dwayne (The Rock) Johnson demonstrated the "Pec Pop of Love." Repeatedly flexing his giant chest muscles alternately over and over, Johnson advised his teenage companion that this move has worked to attract women for thousands of years.

Well, guess what? I am now an expert at performing the Pec Pop of Love.

I haven't demonstrated it for my boys because that would totally gross them out. But since I don't have soft breast tissue and my muscles are right under my skin like a man's, I can pop my pecs almost as impressively as The Rock.

This gives Corey and me a good laugh sometimes, but the fact that my body can do this weird thing leads to awkward situations in public. You see, when I get cold, my chest muscles start twitching. So when it's fifty degrees and windy and I'm standing outside at a tennis meet, quietly cheering my boy on (because you don't yell at tennis meets), my muscles move without my blessing. I'm quietly clapping and whispering, "Way to go, Carter," while my boobs spontaneously pec pop away. Thankfully, my layers of clothing generally cover up the evidence, but that doesn't stop me from being self-conscious.

I'm even more self-conscious at my biweekly exercise class at our local rec center. I joined this class in order to regain some strength after my year of cancer, but I didn't anticipate the uneasiness my chest would cause me. My breasts do not move the way other women's breasts move. When we lift weights or do any sort of exercise that relies heavily on my chest muscles, I try to angle myself away from people the best that I can because I'm fearful of what people will think when they see my boobs moving in ways boobs aren't supposed to move.

Women who have over-the-muscle implants or who undergo flap

surgeries don't have this strange consequence of reconstruction. Flap surgeries result in natural breast movement, and though over-the-muscle implants are firmer than natural breasts, they move relatively naturally as well.

A Boob Job, in Comparison

Since women who have undergone breast augmentation retain their breast tissue, and most of the time their muscles still cling to their chest wall, they do not have issues with movement that women who have undergone breast reconstruction have.

Thoughts from a Plastic Surgery Nurse

I've described many differences from a physical perspective between breast reconstruction and breast augmentation, but a nurse's perspective offers clear disparities in the appointments for the two surgeries. Jess, a registered nurse who spent some of her career working in plastic surgery, says these differences are vast.

During an initial consult, both reconstruction and augmentation patients are asked similar questions, but responses are remarkably different. For instance, many women in for a breast augmentation consult don't remember the date of their last mammogram. For these women, a mammogram is just a necessary evil to check off a yearly female to-do list.

But when a mammogram leads to a cancer diagnosis, the story is significantly different. Women tend to remember the day they found out they might have breast cancer. Most often, they also remember the date of their ultrasound, biopsy, and every other event that marked the path to their diagnosis. Dramatic life events tend to sear themselves into our memory banks.

Jess also often saw augmentation patients only once before their surgery, so she didn't develop a relationship with them, but she was deeply affected by some of the reconstruction patients she served. Since women undergoing reconstruction often visit the plastic surgeon's office regularly for months, nurses tend to become emotionally attached.

"I would go home and pray for many of these women. I wasn't prepared for the emotional toll it would take on me as a nurse," Jess said. "And even if I couldn't feel exactly what each of these women was feeling or thinking or going through, I was inspired by them."[7]

Extending Grace to the Tactless

People will stay stupid things to you throughout your reconstruction process. Guaranteed. On my saddest days, I didn't even go out in public because I didn't know if I could emotionally handle whatever hurtful thing I might hear that day. You just do what you've got to do to get through each day, and sometimes that means sending your hubby to the grocery store so you don't have to listen to the checker's story of how her aunt died of cancer last year.

But I have learned something about people who say insensitive and ignorant things. Most of them are not trying to be jerks. They just want to enter your world, but they don't understand how to do it appropriately. So we can choose to get mad (which I definitely did sometimes) and hold a grudge, or we can step into their shoes and remind ourselves that we're not perfect either. I too have said stupid things from time to time when I've misunderstood another person's journey. When I haven't lived that person's pain.

In fact, when I think about that person who was excited for me that I was going to get a boob job, I'm convinced she was just looking for the silver lining. She'd never been exposed to breast reconstruction. She knew nothing of the numbness, the discomfort, and the scars. She wanted to encourage me, not hurt me.

It may sound a little weird, but it helps me to actually stop and silently say things like, "She doesn't understand; God help me forgive her," when I am hit with a comment that takes my breath away. I don't always immediately forgive that person and want to be their best friend, but I have grown in this thing called grace—this giving to others the benefit of the doubt and extending forgiveness when it is not requested.

It's not easy, but it is freeing to forgive and move on. To "let it go" as that annoying Disney song repeats over and over. When I can keep myself from judging a person by his or her comment, I am free to live without the encumbrance of bitterness, anger, and defeat.

And maybe, at some point down the road, I will have the opportunity to gently advise some of those people who make boob job comments of better ways to relate to breast cancer patients so they don't inadvertently make someone else want to throat-punch them.

Note: In this chapter, I explained some key terms and took you on a walk through the day-to-day realities of living with reconstructed breasts. You will find a (non-exhaustive) glossary of medical procedures and implant materials in the back of this book.

Resources

1. Ludwig, Jessica, RN. Email message to author. Ames, Iowa, April 6, 2017.

2. "Breast Augmentation Guide." American Board of Cosmetic Surgery, accessed December 2, 2019. https://www.americanboardcosmeticsurgery.org/procedure-learning-center/breast/breast-augmentation-guide/.

3. "Sensation and Sensation Changes." Loftus Plastic Surgery Center, accessed December 2, 2019. https://infoplasticsurgery.com/?breast/augmentation/risks/sensation.

4. Perdikis, Galen, MD. "A New National Study Will Access Microsurgery Reinnervation." Vanderbilt University Medical Center, July 3, 2019. https://discover.vumc.org/2019/07/resensation-after-breast-reconstruction/.

5. Swanson, Eric. 2013. "Prospective Outcome Study of 225 Cases of Breast Augmentation." *Plastic and Reconstructive Surgery* 131, no 5: 1158–66. https://journals.lww.com/plasreconsurg/Abstract/2013/05000/Prospective_Outcome_Study_of_225_Cases_of_Breast.45.aspx.

6. West, Diana. "Breastfeeding after Breast Augmentation Surgery." BFAR Information and Support, accessed December 2, 2019. https://www.bfar.org/possible-augmentation.shtml.

7. Jessica Ludwig, email message to author.

Chapter 4

Be Your Own Advocate: Nobody Knows Your Body Better Than You

"Asking for what you need, what you want, and what you're worth requires practice. So practice self-love and start asking."
—Ann Marie Houghtailing

"That's where we film our porn."

Those words actually came out of my first plastic surgeon's mouth. While I sat on the exam table half-naked and fearing for my life, he made a porn joke. (This is the guy I mentioned briefly in Chapter 1. From here on out, he will be known as Dr. Playboy.)

After that comment, he laughed at himself, gave a little flip of his wiry gray hair, and asked me to stand in front of a big blue screen so my cancerous boobs could be photographed. For medical purposes, of course. But after that comment I was more than a little freaked out about what he does with these photos on the side.

I was stressed out even before I entered Dr. Playboy's office. Corey and I were told to be there twenty minutes in advance, but we were given the wrong address. We found ourselves driving around an unfamiliar part of the city as our GPS led us to an ominous abandoned building. By the time we made it to the real office, we were late. The waiting room, complete with a mirrored ceiling framed by neon lights, made me feel like I'd walked into a mash-up episode of *Miami Vice* and *The Jetsons*. I hoped this address was also wrong.

It wasn't.

I tried to be open-minded while I sat in that time-warp waiting room, but it was hard. *Maybe this guy will be okay. He might just be really into disco.* But it felt more likely that he enjoyed spending his spare time in the presence of women with short skirts and big boobs.

After a long, uncomfortable wait, Corey and I were ushered into a small exam room where I was told to remove my shirt, put on a pink paper vest open to the front, and wait for the doctor. That wasn't out of the ordinary. I was getting used to the *open to the front* routine.

Dr. Playboy came in, and I took off my vest to be examined. He agreed with my general surgeon's recommendation that because of the small size of my breasts and the placement of the tumor, a mastectomy really was the best option. Then he proceeded with the rest of the appointment without giving my vest back. Those vests are not my favorite, but they sure do beat being topless. I sat uncomfortably on the exam table while he told me about the procedure he planned to use. He laid it all out there using phrases like "state-of-the-art" and "we'll take good care of you." All while I sat topless. The guy bragged about his experience and skills while I shivered and tried desperately to hold back tears.

I just want to put a shirt on. Does this guy realize I have cancer? Does he understand that I'm not in here for a boob job? That I didn't choose this? Can I just crawl into the cabinet in the corner and die of humiliation?

That Twilight Zone appointment preceded a surgery-scheduling session that wasn't much better. We went to an office where a woman who appeared to have utilized the plastic surgeon's enhancement services sat behind a desk. The woman in the very low-cut V-neck told me that the doctor's first available surgery date was six weeks later.

What??? Hey, lady, did you catch the fact that I have cancer growing in my body? Can you maybe slide me in ahead of a few boob jobs?

Corey and I were so anxious to get out of there that we just scheduled for the first available surgery date and left. On the way home, I cried. I cried because I felt helpless. I cried because I was scared. I cried because a doctor who was supposed to help me made a porn joke while taking photos of my boobs. What kind of bizarre world had I entered?

Advocating for the Best Medical Personnel

Corey and I both felt seriously uneasy about Dr. Playboy, but we weren't sure what to do. When I got home, I called both my family doctor (whom I love dearly) and my friend who walked the cancer road with her daughter. Both of them told me to request a new surgeon. In fact, my friend who realized it was almost 4:00 p.m. while we talked said, "We are going to hang up right now because you need to call the general surgeon before his office closes and ask for a different referral."

So I did.

I felt a little bad about it though. Like I should have just sucked it up and been okay with Dr. Playboy. But I wasn't okay with it. Not one bit okay. And I've learned through my breast reconstruction experience that it is OKAY to not be okay with all the decisions medical professionals make, or even to look elsewhere if they don't fit the type of care you'd like to receive.

My refusal to return to Dr. Playboy's office was my first experience with self-advocacy in the medical world. Ellen Stovall, cancer survivor and National Center for Cancer Survivorship President and CEO, and Elizabeth Johns Clark, PhD, MSW, say this in regard to self-advocacy:

Advocacy for yourself may be the difference that turns feeling hopeless and helpless into feeling hopeful. Stated in another way, self-advocacy is a synonym for what some might otherwise call "control" or "empowerment." Self-advocacy implies strength, both physical and mental. Self-advocacy requires participation in the decision-making process. Given our tremendous access to resources for information and support today, a self-advocate need not go to a medical provider and say, "What would you do," or "I'm in your hands," or "just cure me."[1]

I began to learn the truth of Stovall's and Clark's words. I grew up doing what doctors told me to do. Taking the medicines they prescribed. Going to the specialists they recommended. I believed that because they are the professionals, they know what's best for me. But my breast cancer experience taught me that *I* know *me* better than anyone else. I am the only one who can truly speak up for what I need. And just because someone is a doctor, it doesn't mean he or she has all the right answers. As Stovall and Clark said, I did feel more hopeful once I chose to stand up for my own needs.

Corey and I were pleasantly surprised when we walked into the waiting room of plastic surgeon number two. From here on out, I'll call him Dr. Nice. It was a pleasant waiting area with soft recessed lighting. No mirrors. No neon lights. Just beige chairs and magazine-covered side tables. We both felt instantly at ease and sat down to play a friendly game of Trivia Crack on our phones while we waited.

When I entered Dr. Nice's exam room, I was handed another pink paper vest to put on (*open to the front*, of course) and then waited for the doctor to arrive. He walked in with a smile and a handshake, and I immediately felt cared for and important. I had to remove the vest for the breast examination and those dang photos, but immediately afterward he gave it back. For the remainder of the appointment while we discussed options, I sat unexposed. I was comfortable enough to focus on what he was saying, and he didn't brag about all of his accolades and degrees. He was kind and knowledgeable and presented me with a folder filled with additional information and a phone number to call the office if I had any questions.

Where Dr. Playboy acted like he was doing me a huge favor by taking on my surgery, Dr. Nice made me feel like we were a team. He knew what he thought was the best plan moving forward, but he wanted me to be on board with him.

Not everything about Dr. Nice was perfect. He was a little oblivious to the physical pain involved with gradually filling chest expanders. He liked to use words like "uncomfortable" instead of "excruciating," and he said things like, "Oh, you'll get so used to these that you'll hardly notice they're in there." He'd obviously never had hard saline-filled expanders underneath his chest muscles. But because I knew he genuinely cared about me and about making my breasts look as normal as possible, I overlooked his few flaws.

During this process, it's important to understand that doctors aren't perfect and that they can't read our minds. Most of them appreciate a patient who isn't afraid to ask questions. For those of us enduring breast reconstruction, this process is a significant chapter in our life story. For our doctors and surgeons, it is one of many life stories they are charged with entering into for a short time. *You* know *you*, and he or she needs your input. Finding the confidence to give it is key to achieving the best possible outcome.

Over the course of six months, I had a dozen or more appointments and two surgeries with Dr. Nice. If I did not have the guts to advocate for myself at the beginning, I would have been a wreck in Dr. Playboy's hands.

Another survivor I've talked with, Rachel, had a similar need to advocate for different medical staff. Her mom died of breast cancer when she was in college, and after an aunt was also diagnosed with breast cancer, Rachel tested for the BRCA1 and BRCA2 gene mutation.

Rachel's experience with the genetic counselor she was referred to was pretty awful. Because she had the results of her aunt's gene mutation test in hand, the genetic counselor should have been able to quickly compare Rachel's results to her aunt's. But what took only a week for her sister going through the same process in another state took a month for Rachel. Her genetic counselor was slow to respond to her phone calls, she refused to draw her blood sample on her first visit, and she couldn't find the testing kit on her second visit. Rachel felt frustrated and undervalued as a patient. And when she finally received her results (she was positive for the BRCA2 gene mutation), she couldn't stand the thought of continuing her treatment at that clinic.

She asked for a different referral, and it was one of the best moves she made throughout the mastectomy and reconstruction process.

"Everyone from there on out was so attentive and wonderful and quick to take care of my needs. I can't imagine what it would've been like if I would have stayed at [the original clinic]."

By advocating for herself, Rachel set herself up for success throughout her months of treatment.

Advocating for Physical and Mental Well-Being

Sleeping after my bilateral mastectomy and first phase of reconstructive surgery was challenging. The physical pain that always comes from major trauma to the body was difficult to deal with at the start. But even after that pain left, sleep eluded me. I had expanders in my chest for months. They were rock-hard and tended to pinch on the outside of my breast when I tried to lie on my side. So I was forced to become a back sleeper. I wasn't able to sleep for more than two to three hours at a time and regularly found myself zoning out to Netflix in the wee hours of the morning. Exhaustion became the rule of the day, sleeplessness the rule of the night.

After a couple months of this torture, I finally asked my plastic surgeon if he would prescribe something to help me sleep. I didn't like his response.

"I don't like sleeping pills. They leave you groggy for hours in the morning." He refused to prescribe a sleeping aid for me simply because he personally didn't like the way they made him feel. He assured me that I would get used to it. At that point I wanted to punch him (and this is Dr. Nice I'm talking about).

When I got home, at Corey's urging, I made a call to my beloved family doctor who prescribed an amazing little pill that gave me my sanity back. Sleep returned. I still woke up during the night, and I still really wanted to roll over on my side or tummy, but the pill relaxed me enough that I could drift back to sleep on my backside.

If I hadn't advocated for myself in this area, my family would have suffered. A sleepless mama is not a good mama. And a sleepless wife is not a good wife. When I started sleeping at night, my patience improved, healthy thoughts increased, and pretty much every part of my daily routine got better. Exhaustion makes everything harder. Frustration comes quicker. Impatience wins out over compassion. Unhealthy thought patterns win out over logical thought patterns. (And when you have cancer, it is so easy to slide down the slippery slope of bad thoughts.) I can hardly even put into words how much better I felt when I was no longer sleep starved—when I became a fully functioning wife and mom again.

I learned from my experience, but one of survivor Rachel's regrets is not asking for something to help her sleep. Her body, like mine, fought sleep every night, but she was uneasy asking for sleeping pills because she was concerned she might become addicted. So she just waited it out and dealt with the lack of sleep.

"In hindsight, I wish I would have asked for sleeping pills. I've learned that everything in life is easier to handle when you get the sleep you need. I would've handled the emotions of it better if I had been getting sleep."

Stovall and Clark say that advocacy can improve your quality of life.[2] I wholeheartedly agree. I found it to be true in the arena of sleep. Another survivor, Cathy, found she had to ask for what she needed in the arena of physical therapy.

Some plastic surgeons refer all of their breast reconstruction patients to a physical therapist as part of their routine treatment, and some don't. Dr. Nice didn't, and I got by with some advice from my physical therapist sister-in-law. The exercises she gave me to do at home improved my range of motion.

Cathy, on the other hand, felt strongly that she needed to visit a physical therapist even though her surgeon didn't initially offer her a referral. She took the initiative and asked her surgeon for a referral, which he agreed to do.

"It was so beneficial. Crawling my fingers up the wall like my surgeon suggested just wasn't working," she said. "The physical therapist manipulated my arm and it got stronger a lot faster than it would've on my own."

Cathy's physical therapist also worked on her tummy where she had a hip-to-hip incision from her **DIEP flap reconstruction surgery** (reconstruction that utilizes abdominal body tissue instead of implants). He pushed and twisted on the scarred area, keeping the scar tissue from building up underneath the skin. It was an unexpected benefit from her physical therapy sessions.

"Who knows what my tummy would look like now if I hadn't had the physical therapy treatment," she said. "It was torture, but it was worth it."

Our physical and mental well-being are worth advocating for, and sometimes finding the courage to stand up for what we need gives us even greater benefits than we expect.

Advocating for the Type of Surgery You Want

There are a lot of different types and stages of breast cancer, and there are diverse types of surgeries women can undergo during their course of treatment. Your general surgeon or plastic surgeon may recommend something that you just can't get on board with. It is okay to question him or her about the recommendations.

Self-advocacy played a major role in treatment with survivor Amber when she was diagnosed with stage III breast cancer. Her surgeon assumed she wanted to have a bilateral mastectomy. But from the moment she found out she had cancer, Amber knew she wanted to keep as much of her natural body as she could. She questioned in her mind whether or not she should ask about a single mastectomy. She ultimately decided that it was worth talking to her surgeon about keeping her cancer-free breast.

The surgeon was quick to tell her that it was 100 percent her decision to make. He showed her stats and figures to help with her decision, and she was confident in her choice to do a single instead of a bilateral. He also pointed out that if she chose a single and later had regrets, she could have another surgery to remove the remaining native breast. But if she went with bilateral surgery and had regrets, there was no going back.

She then talked to her oncologist, who was also supportive and told her, "You do whatever it is you need to do to help you sleep at night. If you have peace of mind doing a single mastectomy, do it. It's entirely up to you."

The pendulum seems to swing in the mastectomy department. When Cathy had her single mastectomy seventeen years ago, the option for a bilateral wasn't even mentioned to her. Today, bilateral mastectomies are very common. Many women choose to have both breasts removed for their peace of mind, even when cancer has not been found in the opposite breast.

I knew from the get-go that I wanted to have both breasts removed. I figured that boobs are not necessary for life, and if they were gone I wouldn't have to worry about cancer coming back on the opposite side. Like Amber's doctor said, "You do whatever is going to help you sleep at night."

I don't regret my decision, but I have found that I really do miss my breasts. They were small and not so pretty, but they had feeling in them. And they were a natural piece of me. I'm used to the numbness for the most part, but I miss the sensation. I miss that part of me that is forever gone.

This is a tough decision, and different surgeons and oncologists have varying opinions, but it is worth thinking about what you really want. Have a collaborative discussion with your doctors before following their recommendations blindly.

Advocating for Information

Seeking information is a key part of self-advocacy. Attaining as much knowledge as you can about your medical condition and possible treatment options puts you in the driver's seat, less likely to be swayed by recommendations that make you uncomfortable.

This was the case for me, as I chose not to undergo nipple reconstruction, which means my boobs are smooth across the front. I did, however, opt for tattooing so they would look a little more "normal." But I knew nothing about medical tattooing, and I wanted to know what a tattooed nipple would look like. Tattoos are permanent, and even though I knew very few people would ever see my tattoos, I wanted them to look good. I really wanted to see some photos of Dr. Nice's aestheticist's (tattoo artist's) work before getting inked. What if they looked terrible? There would be no way to erase them once I had them done.

It was surprisingly difficult to get an appointment to look at photos. I knew the clinic had them. They took "before" photos of me, so I was certain they had "finished product" photos as well. It felt so weird to call the medical clinic to ask if I could schedule an appointment to look at photos of nipple tattoos, but I knew I could not go forward without more information. It took three phone calls to the clinic before I finally received the go-ahead to stop in and look at photos.

I could have just given up and trusted they would be okay, but neither Corey nor I had a settled feeling about doing something major without gathering all the information we could. We were pleasantly surprised by how real many of the tattoos looked. If I crossed my eyes a little, I almost couldn't tell they weren't the real thing. That put Corey's mind and my own at ease for my tattoo appointment, which made it completely worth the nagging I had to do.

Like my persistence in calling the doctor's office, survivor Amber had to push for information on breast size after reconstruction, and she never felt like she got a full picture of reconstructed breast sizing compared to natural breast sizing.

"They talked in cc's (cubic centimeters), and that didn't make sense to me. And they never gave me a book to look at or even asked how large I wanted to be."

Because Amber had a single mastectomy, her doctors assumed she wanted to match her new breast to her remaining natural breast size and shape. But what she really wanted was a reduction. She knew they would be performing a surgery on the natural breast to tweak it anyway, and she wanted that to include reducing size. But no one asked her what she wanted.

She decided she had to make it clear to her surgeon that she wanted smaller breasts. Once she broached the subject, he was on board with her wishes. But if she hadn't brought it up, he wouldn't have asked.

It can be hard to advocate for ourselves. We tend to assume that doctors know best and are often tempted to follow their suggestions blindly. But doctors are people just like us. They make mistakes. They have opinions that are often developed from a worldview different from our own. They may even get stuck in a rut and just do with you what they do with other patients because "that's what they do."

But your body is your body. And *you* know *you* better than anyone else. The quality of your breast reconstruction experience is greatly impacted when you become an educated, proactive advocate for your own medical care. It definitely impacted mine. (See the sidebars for Self-Advocacy Pointers and Stovall and Clark's list of reasons for self-advocacy.)

Self-Advocacy Pointers

- Research your plastic surgeon's background; this is so easy to do in the world of the internet. Look up your surgeon, and if possible, find some of their patients and ask them about their experience. When I was referred to my second plastic surgeon, I found a "getting to know you" video of him online and was immediately put at ease because he seemed so normal.
- Research the treatments your doctor suggests and come back with questions before settling on a course of action. Are they recommending silicone when you think you'd feel more comfortable with saline? Do your research and talk to your doctor about it.
- Don't be afraid to ask for a second opinion. We sometimes think we should just listen to the expert sitting across the room from us, but different surgeons do things in different ways and it doesn't hurt to talk to a couple experts before making decisions.
- Go with your gut. I have found my gut to be pretty reliable, and I am so thankful I went with that gut feeling and found a different plastic surgeon. With the amount of time you spend with your plastic surgeon, it is well worth it to have one you like.

Stovall and Clark: Important Reasons for Self-Advocacy[3]

- Advocacy gives you some stability and a feeling of regaining some control in your life.
- Advocacy is confidence building in the way it helps you face challenges that seem insurmountable.
- Advocacy is a way of reaching out to others. It can be as simple as asking your doctor or nurse for the name of someone to talk with who survived your particular type of cancer.
- Advocacy can improve your quality of life.
- Advocacy for yourself may be the difference that turns feeling hopeless and helpless into feeling hopeful. Stated in another way, self-advocacy is a synonym for what some might otherwise call "control" or "empowerment." Self-advocacy implies strength, both physical and mental. Self-advocacy requires participation in the decision-making process. Given our tremendous access to resources for information and support today, a self-advocate need not go to a medical provider and say "What would you do" or "I'm in your hands" or "Just cure me."
- Commitment to shared responsibility with your medical team can contribute to the goal of valuable physical, emotional, and mental health.

Resources

1. "Becoming a Self-Advocate." National Coalition for Cancer Survivorship, accessed December 2, 2019. https://www.canceradvocacy. org/resources/advocating-for-yourself/becoming-a-self-advocate-2/.
2. Ibid.
3. Ibid.

Chapter 5

Vignettes from the Hospital: Women Share Their Post-Mastectomy Stories

"You're braver than you believe, stronger than you seem, and smarter than you think."
—A. A. Milne

The thought of writing about what to expect after surgery is very intimidating. I want to provide you with encouragement and practical advice, but how do I include all the possible outcomes when there are so many variations to mastectomy and breast reconstruction surgeries and procedures, each with its own unique challenges? How can I write this chapter without leaving something out? The answer is, I can't. And even if I could, no doubt between the minute I hit send on my final draft of this book and the day it hits the bookstores, new developments in reconstruction will occur.

If you are seeking detailed information on all the latest research, procedures, and recovery times, you will not find it here. (Check out the resource section in the back of this book for websites that offer up-to-date breast surgery information.) Instead, in this chapter I will share stories from women who've undergone a variety of procedures, and I'll give you some tips to make your hospital stay easier. But keep in mind, we are all different. We each have different levels of pain tolerance, and our bodies don't heal on a specific universal timetable.

Lengths of hospital stays also vary depending on the type of surgery. A two-night hospital stay is pretty typical for women who've undergone bilateral mastectomies with either direct-to-implant or two-stage reconstruction, and a one-night stay might suffice for someone who has undergone a single mastectomy with either of those types of reconstruction. For women who undergo flap reconstruction, the hospital stay is significantly longer, with an average of five days.[1]

Though your experience will be unique to you, I hope these stories will give you some insight and encouragement as you walk through this very hard thing.

Kim (Me)

Bilateral mastectomy and first phase of implant reconstruction with expanders

"Ten."

When I woke up in the recovery room and the nurse asked me to rate my pain on a scale from one to ten, I said ten. I've been told that number should be reserved for women in childbirth, but I've birthed three children, and I believe the pain of having your boobs amputated is equally deserving of the number. The nurse quickly administered pain medication, and that number dropped to about a five.

When I arrived in my hospital room, I was given this great little button connected to a tube that injected pain meds into my body. I could push it whenever I needed to dim the pain. I soon discovered, however, that though it relieved the pain in my chest, it made my tummy feel like I'd taken one too many rides on the Tilt-a-Whirl. Because of this, my pain med pump was removed and I was at the nurse's bidding for receiving pain relief. This posed quite a problem for me on a couple shifts. Before surgery, I sought advice from women who had gone through this before me, and every one of them told me to make sure to stay ahead of the pain. *Don't be afraid to use your pain meds. That's what they're there for. You don't have to be Superwoman.* This is the advice I received.

But when forced to rely on a nursing staff with too many patients on their roster and their own ideas about how much pain you *should* be experiencing, staying on top of the pain was not easy. One nurse (I will call her Nurse Meanie from here on out) waited until I was on the brink of insanity before giving me pain meds. Her two shifts were definitely the longest of my two-night stay. More than once Corey walked to the nurses' station because she didn't respond to my call. At one point, I was in so much pain that I threw up. My little vomiting episode happened right after shift change, so a poor sweet nurse who'd just arrived on the scene had to start his shift by cleaning up my mess.

"Why did you wait so long for your pain meds?" he asked after I sat in a fresh, clean gown and bed sheets. That simple question was so vindicating. I only wish I would've thrown up right on Nurse Meanie, who told me to hold off on the meds because I "should be tolerating the pain better by now."

I had several different nurses over the course of my stay, and you will too. Some will be better than others. Some have excellent bedside manners and make you feel loved and cared for. Others make you feel about as important as the number on your door. Unfortunately, we don't get to choose who takes care of us in the hospital.

The pain was the worst part for me, but hindered movement also made my hospital stay challenging. A relentlessly itchy nose (a side effect of anesthesia) that I could not reach to scratch my first night in the hospital was almost unbearable. Thank God for my sweet husband who pulled a recliner right up to the side of my bed and stayed with me all night. He held my hand in his, only releasing his grip to scratch that stupid itch on my nose every time I asked.

Claustrophobia hits when you can't move your upper body. And it wasn't just about scratching my nose. I couldn't sit up on my own. I couldn't roll over or switch positions. I could only move my arms from the elbow down. My butt kept getting numb, and Corey had to help me move to relieve the numbness. Needless to say, neither of us slept much that night. It was the first of many, many sleepless nights.

When the morning after surgery day dawned, I felt like crap, with Nurse Meanie back on duty. She told me I needed to walk the halls before they would consider releasing me, and I thought, *What the heck? I don't even want to go home today. Just leave me alone.* But I did eventually get out of bed and walk to the door of the room and back. It felt like an amazing feat. Later that day my body figured out how to pee again. Life was looking up. I started to want to go back to my own home where I could sit on my recliner and take pain meds as needed instead of at the whim of Nurse Meanie. I checked things off the list of necessary accomplishments to receive release papers.

By the time I was released on day two post-surgery, I was able to walk quite a distance down the hall and back. I could even lean my head forward enough to reach the hand holding my toothbrush. Sweet freedom! I could pee, walk, and brush my teeth. I was ready to go home.

Amber

Single mastectomy and first phase of implant reconstruction with expanders

"When I woke up [from surgery] I was like, 'Is it done?' It was weird. I had no pain. And I really didn't have much pain through the whole recovery process."

It relieved Amber to experience minimal pain after her surgery. After undergoing months of chemo, she found that surgery was one of the easier parts of her treatment. She had very little pain in recovery and was back home within twenty-four hours.

"It felt weird not to have pain. I was expecting pain, but I would classify what I experienced as discomfort. The only pain I really felt was from my drains."

Amber was up using the bathroom and brushing her teeth on her own the night of the surgery. She used the pain pump when she felt like she was starting to hurt because, like me, many people encouraged her beforehand to stay ahead of the pain, but she didn't have to rely on pain meds nearly as much as she expected.

For Amber, a later surgery on her native breast to match her newly reconstructed breast was more painful than the mastectomy and reconstruction. That surgery was a **lollipop lift** (where the surgeon cuts around the areola and straight down, allowing him to reshape and move the nipple and areola), and it was a lot more intense than Amber expected.

"When it's all said and done, I'm glad that I had it done. But if I'd known from the get-go, I don't know if I would have made the same decision [about the lollipop lift surgery]."

Rachel

Bilateral mastectomy and first phase of implant reconstruction with expanders

"The first thing I remember thinking after waking up from surgery is, 'I can't get my breath. I can't breathe.'"

When Rachel came out of anesthesia feeling like an elephant sat on her chest, she was terrified. The pain and heaviness felt so intense that she went into panic mode and started crying. "The crying made it hurt even worse. It was excruciating," she said. Her nurses were on the ball and quickly pumped her with meds relieving some of the pain and tightness.

After the initial scare, her hospital experience went pretty smoothly, though she struggled with the pain caused by even the slightest movement. She said, "I didn't realize it was going to hurt like it did. I didn't realize how much I used my chest muscles until every little movement hurt."

This hindered movement took Rachel by surprise. The inability to sit up or comb her hair or brush her teeth was something she hadn't thought about prior to surgery. And her first trip to the bathroom with the night nurse was her most humbling hospital experience. She thought, *What is going on? I can't even sit on the toilet by myself.*

Like my nurse, one of Rachel's doctors mentioned releasing her to go home after one night in the hospital. "I looked at him and thought, *Are you out of your mind? I can't even walk down the hall and you want me to go home?*"

Rachel did stay a second night and felt more ready to head out into the world the next day.

Judi

DIEP flap reconstruction to replace silicone implants

"My first thought coming out of anesthesia was how incredibly hot I was!"

Some surgeons request the recovery room temperature be kept extra warm because cooler temps can restrict blood flow. Once Judi was in her own room and at a more comfortable temperature, her time in the hospital went better than expected, which she believes was due in part to **guided meditation** (meditation in response to someone else's guidance through a variety of possible means, like in person, video, audio, or written text). A therapist introduced her to guided meditation prior to surgery, and she spent time listening to a relaxing meditation twice a day for a few months leading up to her surgery. The day of surgery, the hospital staff agreed to her request to play a meditation CD as she went under anesthesia and as she came out of it.

She said, "I was skeptical of the studies that showed that people [who practiced guided meditation] didn't need as much pain medication, but somehow it worked for me." Judi was able to switch from strong prescription medications to Tylenol after the first forty-eight hours. She thinks it was due to a combination of guided meditation and an **ON-Q* pain pump** (a type of pain relief system that utilizes a pump ball connected to a tube that's inserted at the surgical site, continuously delivering local anesthesia to block the pain in the area of the procedure).

Judi spent a full five days in the hospital, which is pretty typical for DIEP surgery because of the intensity of the procedure.

Misty

Bilateral mastectomy and first phase of reconstruction with expanders

"They put me on the maternity floor."

After Misty's bilateral mastectomy and first phase of reconstruction, the hospital floor she should have stayed on was full, so she was assigned to the maternity floor. She received many "Congratulations" from well-meaning strangers who had no idea that she was not, in fact, a celebratory new mom but a brokenhearted young woman with breast cancer.

"As I walked the halls, people always congratulated me. That was the hardest thing. It got to the point that I had to just thank them and move on," she said.

And it wasn't just misplaced congratulations that made Misty uncomfortable—it was the nurses who didn't know quite what to do with her. The labor and delivery nurses were unfamiliar with mastectomy and breast reconstruction protocol. She said, "The nurses weren't trained to handle me. They had me up and walking the halls too soon for a mastectomy patient, and they didn't understand my limited arm movement, so they'd leave my food too far away to reach."

In addition, one nurse performed a big no-no by placing ice

packs on her chest. Misty's surgery was nipple-sparing, and when you keep your nipples they need good blood flow to remain healthy. The restricted blood flow to the nipples when iced puts them at risk of dying. Thankfully, her plastic surgeon discovered the ice faux pas before it caused any damage.

Emily

Left breast (right was done in a previous surgery) mastectomy and DIEP flap reconstruction on both sides

"I've never had pain like the pain I had in my abdomen those first two days after surgery."

Emily experienced mild pain in her chest after her DIEP flap, but it was nothing compared to the pain in her abdomen. She later developed **hematomas** (blood clots that form in the tissues, outside of the blood vessel) in her breasts, which were extremely painful and required two more surgeries, but during her initial hospital stay for DIEP, the abdominal pain was overwhelming.

Emily took full advantage of the IV pain medication prescribed to her at the hospital. The pain in her abdomen was so agonizing that she nearly screamed and might have said some bad words when the nurse helped her sit up and get to the bathroom. "I'm pretty sure I swore a few times, but I apologized."

In addition to the pain, Emily also struggled with the fact that she had to humble herself and let her family help her due to her limited mobility. But she found it actually ended up being a blessing. "I'm a very independent person, but being forced to let [my mom and sister] help me made me feel closer to them in some strange way. My mom kissed my forehead once while I was in the hospital and she hasn't kissed me ever in my life. That I remember."

Darci

DIEP flap surgery (bilateral mastectomy with insertion of expanders was completed in a previous surgery)

"It was almost traumatic, it hurt so much."

The act of being moved from one bed to another after her release from the ICU was one of the most painful experiences of Darci's life. She was moved out of the ICU because she was doing well, but that good news didn't make the transition easy. In addition to the initial pain of being positioned in her new bed, every little body movement hurt. "Everything I tried to move caused a good amount of pain. You cough, it hurts. You laugh, it hurts. You try to move your arm to grab something, it hurts."

Many women who undergo DIEP flap spend the first night or two in the ICU. Newly attached blood vessels need almost constant observation to make sure they are functioning properly. **Doppler probe (Doppler blood flow) monitors** (an implantable ultrasound probe attached to a wire that leads from the reattached blood vessels to the outside of the body, where it is connected to a monitor that keeps track of blood flow) are inserted during DIEP flap and are used to make sure the blood is flowing through the newly attached vessels. Darci said the doctors checked her monitors every hour for a full twenty-four hours and then kept watching closely for the duration of her hospital stay. "I was told seventy-two hours was a magic number for the blood vessels because at that point, a kind of tissue or membrane has formed to start the healing process."

Darci spent five days in the hospital after her DIEP flap, and each day she received a new goal to complete in regard to movement. She sat in a chair (albeit not comfortably) within thirty-six hours of surgery and started taking short walks the following day. By the time she was released to go home, the pain was very manageable, and she was able to wean herself from prescription pain meds within a week.

Tips for Your Hospital Stay

As you can see, the hospital recovery experience varies from woman to woman, depending on body types, pain tolerance, the type of surgery, and even what hospital floor you are assigned to. But regardless of the specifics of the experience, the hospital stay is generally no walk in the park. The following are some helpful hints for your hospital recovery:

Have Someone Stay with You

If it's not realistic to have one person take on the entire hospital stay with you, I recommend divvying up those hospital hours. Prior to surgery, make a schedule and ask your friends and family to take shifts to stay with you. You will find that having a support person present is invaluable. I don't know what I would have done without Corey there to check in at the nurse's station when no one responded to my call. And how would I have survived the night with my sanity intact without him by my side repeatedly scratching my itchy nose?

Stay Ahead of the Pain

Regardless of what Nurse Meanie thinks, keeping your pain under control is a very good thing. And if one pain medication isn't working or makes you feel nauseous, let your nurse or doctor know. There are so many different pain meds they can prescribe to you. It's not worth it to put up with a pain med that's not working the way you think it should. And your body will heal more quickly if you are comfortable.[2]

Be Self-Aware

If the hospital staff tries to push you out the door before you are ready to go, don't be afraid to advocate for yourself. On the other hand, if you feel ready to go home before they plan to release you, don't be afraid to make that known too. It can be intimidating to stand up for yourself when you feel like the doctors and nurses should know best, but nobody knows your body better than you do.

It's Okay to Say No Visitors

If you don't want visitors, don't be afraid to say so. I knew beforehand that I would not want visitors while in the hospital. This felt like such an intimate surgery, and I read up on the pain I would likely experience after the anesthesia wore off. I didn't want to deal with people on top of the pain, so Corey sent out a mass email requesting no visitors at the hospital. I don't regret that decision one bit. Only family and very close friends were allowed in my hospital room, which gave me the time I needed to rest and recover while avoiding the awkwardness of unwanted visitors.

Bring Some Comforts from Home

It's amazing what a little something from home will do to make you more comfy in the hospital. Super soft socks with nonskid soles were my favorite bring-from-home item. They not only felt fantastic on my feet, but they kept me from sliding around as I walked to the bathroom and up and down the hall. Your own pajamas, a pillow, or even one of your child's stuffed animals may help you feel more at home in unfamiliar surroundings.

Your time in the hospital will definitely not be a relaxing getaway, but you can do it.

Resources

1. "DIEP Flap Reconstruction: What to Expect." Breastcancer.org, updated March 7, 2019. https://www.breastcancer.org/treatment/surgery/reconstruction/types/autologous/diep/what-to-expect.
2. "Mastectomy Surgery Checklist." Facing Our Risk of Cancer Empowered (FORCE), accessed December 2, 2019. https://www.facingourrisk.org/uploads/mastectomy-surgery-checklist.pdf.

Chapter 6

At-Home Recovery: It's Not an Easy Road

"Healing takes courage, and we all have courage. Even
if we have to dig a little to find it."
—Tori Amos

"No one needs a shower this big."

That thought ran through my mind as I unpacked boxes for the
bathroom when we moved into our new house. Seriously, we could
have had a party in that cavernous tiled shower. (But we didn't, because
that would be weird and awkward and just plain wrong.)

About a year later, I had my breasts removed, and that shower went
from an unnecessary luxury to an amazing gift. Some may think it
a lovely coincidence that my family moved into a house with a giant
shower a year before I was diagnosed with breast cancer, but I have
been a believer in Jesus long enough to know that He gives good gifts.
And sometimes those gifts are totally unexpected—and maybe even
a little weird. That shower was one of His weird and perfect gifts.
He knew I would be diagnosed with cancer while living in the house
with the big shower, and He knew that my 6-foot-2-inch 200-pound

husband, a shower chair, and I would all appreciate a little extra elbow room.

I remember my first shower after surgery. Sitting in the shower chair and letting my husband bathe me was one of the most intimate and humbling experiences of my life. It took great effort to walk to the bathroom, stand while he undressed me, and then sit upright under the warm flow of water. By the time I was dry and dressed again, I felt like I'd ran a marathon.

Showering is just one of many hurdles I jumped (maybe "crawled over" is a better description) as I recovered from this major surgery. I'm sure you will also cross over a variety of hurdles in the aftermath of having your breasts removed and reconstructed. I hope the following pages will help you prepare for your recovery.

At-Home Recovery

It's such a relief to be released from the hospital and return home where everything is familiar and nurses and doctors don't poke and prod you at all hours of the day and night. But being home doesn't mean being healed. For many women, it takes several weeks to start feeling normal again.

As with the hospital stay, each woman's at-home recovery experience is different. For instance, you might have surgical drains for seven days after surgery, but maybe you'll still have output at week three. You might have two drains, or maybe you'll have six. You might wean yourself off of prescription medication soon after arriving home, or you might still need it a month later. You might be able to lie on your bed to sleep soon after surgery, or (if you are like me) you'll spend the better part of two months sleeping on a recliner.

Furniture

First of all, plan ahead so that when you return home you can be as comfortable as possible. I spent my first several days at home exclusively in my *recovery recliner*, a loveseat recliner we purchased specifically for my recovery. The only time I left my seat was to go to the bathroom or take short walks up and down the hall. Buying my recovery recliner was far and away the best move we made to make my first days at home more comfortable. Another survivor, Emily, went one step further and (in addition to buying a couch with a power recliner for the living room) purchased a chaise with a reclining back that sat right next to her bed for sleeping at night.

If reclining furniture is not in your budget, consider borrowing a recliner from a friend or family member for a few weeks. Having a comfortable piece of furniture to sleep in at night is vital, and having one in a common area of your house allows you to feel like you are still part of your family's activities, even if you are more of an observer at this point.

Pillows

Pillows will be your friend, especially if you plan to sleep in your bed. I didn't lie flat in bed until after my implant exchange surgery because my expanders were so uncomfortable. Another survivor, Judi, was told by her surgeon not to lie flat on her back for four weeks after DIEP flap surgery. Some women are able to find a comfortable position by using a variety of different shapes and sizes of pillows for support, but you might want to consider purchasing a wedge pillow to sleep on for a while. I bought one and it gave me a second sleeping option. Many times I started out the night in bed on my wedge pillow and then moved to the recliner after a couple hours.

Under-the-knee bolster pillows and mastectomy pillows are also useful. A bolster pillow is especially handy after DIEP flap because it allows you to relax your legs while preventing them from stretching out and pulling at your sore abdomen. Mastectomy pillows come in different shapes and sizes, but their purpose is the same—to relieve pain and pressure caused by your arms hanging flat at your sides.

Some women prefer one large rectangular pillow that wraps all the way from your left side to your right with cutouts for your armpits. Others use two separate pillows, often in the shape of a heart. (*These are available for free at my website, kimharms.net.*)

Drains and Drain Bulbs

During surgery, drain tubes will be placed in your chest. These tubes attach to drain bulbs that hang from your body and serve to remove blood, pus, and other fluids as you heal. They will likely be an extension of your body for at least a week, but two weeks—or even three weeks— isn't out of the question. If you had a bilateral mastectomy with implant reconstruction, you will likely have two drains. If you went the route of flap reconstruction, you will probably have four drains or more. The number varies depending on the individual and the type of surgery.

The drain bulbs need to be emptied regularly, and the amount of liquid must be charted. The volume of discharge varies from person to person, and as you heal, output decreases. (An increase in output is a sign that something might be wrong.) If you are like me, you will not have any desire to empty your own drainage bulbs. I strategically asked my retired nurse mother-in-law to come stay with us for the first few days so she could help with drains if needed.

The drain bulbs and attached tubes are pretty annoying. Mine always felt like they were in the way, and when they accidentally got tugged on it made me want to cuss. Products on the market have been created specifically to contain the drain. I tried a camisole with drain pockets the first day home, but I found it incredibly uncomfortable and nearly impossible to get on and off. The winner for me was a front-zip hoodie with drain pockets sewn inside.

But this was what worked for me. Because of the many different surgeries and body types, a variety of options exist to help you feel more comfortable during your recovery. Expect some trial and error as you discover what you like. I recommend getting a few options to try. For example, Emily started out with some mastectomy T-shirts with drain pockets, but the drains tugged when she wore them. She ultimately bought drain scarves from an Etsy store that tie around the waist, and she loved them. In another case, when Judi first arrived home, she wore her robe inside out and placed the drain bulbs in the pockets. This wasn't as comfortable as she hoped, so she made her own drain pockets and attached them with Velcro to her DIEP compression belly wrap.

Some of these ideas may work for you, or you may come up with other solutions, but it is definitely worthwhile to put some forethought into how you plan to keep all that drain tubing under control.

Pain Control and Constipation

Oxycodone was my friend the first few days at home. I watched the clock closely and often had to bide my time until the next dose because the pain always came back before it was time to medicate. Though the pain relief from Oxycodone was fantastic, I didn't like how it made me sleepy and dazed (and I didn't like the idea of taking something with the potential for addiction), so I weaned myself off of it as quickly as I could. After a week or so on full-strength, I worked to increase the time in between doses and got by with ibuprofen to take the edge off.

In addition to feeling dazed and tired, another unpleasant side effect of many prescription pain meds is constipation. Stool softeners are recommended to fight the constipating effects of pain meds, but when I got through the first week without being constipated, I thought I was in the clear and stopped taking them. Big mistake! About two weeks after surgery, I experienced the worst constipation I have ever had in my life. The pain of the poop was unreal. Don't do that to yourself. Drink tons of water and take the highest dose of stool softeners recommended until you are completely weaned from prescription painkillers. I promise you will not regret it.

Bathing

As I mentioned earlier, bathing is a challenge. Depending on the type of surgery you had and your doctor's recommendation, you may not be allowed to shower for a few days. If this is the case for you, it's nice to have dry shampoo and disposable cleansing wipes on hand. My surgeon gave the okay to shower the day I went home, as long as I was cautious about my incisions and drain areas. I protected my chest by facing away from the water flow as I sat in my shower chair (another item I recommend buying or borrowing), and I attached my drain bulbs to a lanyard around my neck.

Not only do you need to be careful when showering, but you will also likely need help. Corey helped me shower, but if you don't have a hubby to help out, consider which close friend or relative you might ask. It's such a humbling position to be in, but the end result is a clean body . . . and that is refreshing.

Sleep Aids

I was dreadfully tired after surgery, but sleep eluded me. Between the pain, the fact that I couldn't lie down comfortably, my inability to switch positions without help, and those awful drains hanging out of my body, I seriously struggled in the sleep department. I spent many sleep-starved nights in my recovery recliner before I asked my doctor for a prescription for sleeping pills to help save my sanity.

If you can't sleep on your own, get help. Don't try to be Superwoman. Your body needs sleep. Try an over-the-counter sleep aid or ask your doctor about a prescription. I don't know about you, but when I don't sleep, everything I have to deal with in the waking hours is ten times harder, and I can be one grumpy mama. Your body, your mind, and your family will appreciate a mom who gets some rest.

Mobility

Mobility can be one of the most serious challenges when you return home. I remember the effort it took to get from my hospital room to

Corey's truck, and then getting through the thirty-minute drive from Des Moines to Huxley. After I walked into my house and sat down on the recliner, I wondered if I would ever move again.

The act of walking is exhausting, but not being able to move your arms above your head or use your chest muscles (and if you have a DIEP flap, losing the use of your abdominal muscles as well) can make the smallest tasks incredibly difficult. Reaching into a cupboard is nearly impossible without a step stool, and some women find it helpful to have extendable grabbers for retrieving things. Getting in and out of a chair or bed is also a job. Until I regained some strength in my chest, I figured out a way to shimmy to the edge of the recliner seat and then use my leg muscles to get to a standing position. Another survivor, Judi, used leggings in a unique way to help her get in and out of bed after her DIEP flap. She placed a pair across the bed to lie down on, and when she wanted to get up, a family member would take hold of each end of the leggings underneath her and use them to pull her to a sitting position.

Movement can be painful and exhausting, but regular movement is key to recovering well. I was so annoyed when the nurses at the hospital tried to get me to walk before I felt ready. But I remember that when I did, it gave my attitude a boost and made me feel like I accomplished something. You don't have to move far or fast; just make efforts to keep moving. You will eventually go from short trips down the hall to a trip to the mailbox and, soon, a walk around the block. And before long, you will ease back into real-life activities. I was so excited the day I felt good enough to attend one of my son's track meets.

Though not all surgeons refer their mastectomy patients to a physical therapist, Susan Beck, DO, highly recommends her patients go to at least one physical therapy session, even if they don't necessarily want to. She said, "I have noticed as a practicing physician that my patients just get fatigued from appointments. And the one they most readily drop is physical therapy. I always tell my patients, 'Please,

please, please don't give that one up.' There are so many things they can teach you comfort-wise."[1]

Both physical therapy sessions and at-home exercises are helpful to improve your movement in recovery. See the sidebar for at-home stretching suggestions, or contact your physician or physical therapist for exercise options tailored to your specific needs.

Stretching Exercises

Listed below are several post-mastectomy stretching exercises paraphrased from a variety of medical websites. You can find these sites in the recommended resources section at the back of this book. Remember that it's important to follow your surgeon's instructions for exercise. He or she may even have a list of their own suggestions for you.

- **Shoulder Shrugs.** Raise your shoulder toward your ears and try to bring your shoulder blades together in the back. Repeat several times.
- **Shoulder Circles.** Roll small forward circles with your shoulders. Slowly increase the size of the circle. Repeat several times.
- **Wall-Facing Finger Wall Walk.** Stand facing a wall and walk your fingers up the wall. When you get to the point where you feel a stretch, but not pain, stay in that position for ten to fifteen seconds and then walk your fingers back down. Repeat several times.
- **Perpendicular Finger Wall Walk.** Stand perpendicular to the wall so your arm is out to your side, and not in front of you, and walk your fingers up the wall as in the previous exercise. Repeat several times.
- **Forward Arm Lifts.** Lie on your back or sit on a chair with your arms at your side. Lift your arms until

they are above your head. Lower your arms and repeat.

- **Windshield Wipers.** Lie on your back or sit on a chair with your arms at your sides. Bending at the elbow, raise your lower arm up with fingers pointed to the ceiling. Lower your arms and repeat.
- **Snow Angel.** Lie on your back with your arms at your sides and raise your arms over your head and back down to your sides, just like you did in the snow when you were a kid.
- **Trunk Side Bend.** Stand with your legs apart and arms at your side. Lean to one side, sliding your arm down your leg. Return to a standing straight position and repeat on the other side.
- **Clasped-Hand Arm Lifts.** Clasp your hands together in front of your chest with your elbows out. Slowly lift your arms upward until you feel the stretch. Lower arms and repeat.
- **Back Climb.** Clasp your hands behind your back and slowly raise your straight arms up and back down. Repeat.

Lymphedema

Because I had only the **sentinel lymph node** (the first lymph node where cancer will spread from the original tumor site) removed during my surgery, I don't have **lymphedema** (swelling most often caused by the removal of lymph nodes or damage done to lymph nodes during cancer treatment). The more lymph nodes you have removed during surgery, the more likely you are to have lymphedema struggles. The symptoms (which include achiness, heaviness, swelling, decreased flexibility, and tightness) generally occur in the arm, but the hand, underarm, chest wall, and breast can all be affected as well.[2]

Symptoms occur when a blockage in the lymphatic system prevents lymph fluid from draining normally. It often takes time to appear; months or even a few years after you've recovered is not uncommon.[3] If and when lymphedema strikes, call your doctor right away. Though lymphedema is not curable, if treated in early stages the prognosis can improve. Special exercises, compression sleeves, and manual lymphatic drainage (MLD) sessions with a lymphedema therapist are all common forms of treatment.

Helping Hands

As you can see from the topics explored in this chapter, recovering at home is a slow process, and it's not one you should try to handle on your own. Because of limited mobility, it's crucial to have someone available to help you during the day. (See sidebar for areas where you may need help.) Corey works close to home and his boss is pretty awesome, so he was able to be with me any time I needed him. He often came home for lunch to help me shower. But Corey wasn't my only helper. My in-laws also stayed for a week, followed by my mom, who stayed with us off and on for several weeks.

Survivor Darci can attest to the importance of having help during recovery. She lives alone and made plans prior to surgery to have her mom and sister stay with her. When they had to return home, one of her grown daughters came to help. If a friend or relative is unable to help out in this way, consider looking into hiring a home health aide for a short time.

I'm sure I have not covered every possible *returning home* topic in this chapter, but I hope this at least gives you a glimpse of what you might expect in the days and weeks after your breast surgery.

Areas Where You May Need Help

- **Meals.** If possible, arrange a meal schedule for your recovery, or have someone do this for you. We set a large cooler on our front porch so people could simply drop the meal off and leave. If you have time prior to surgery and you feel up to it, make some freezer meals for your recovery. It's likely you have some friends and/or family members who would be happy to make a few freezer meals too.

- **Cleaning.** Your friends probably want to clean your house for you. It's a little humbling to have someone else come scrub your toilets, but let them do it. They are helping you (which is awesome), and by helping you, they feel useful. If having friends or family clean is not an option, you might want to consider hiring a cleaning service a few times during your recovery.

- **Taxiing.** When you first get home, you won't be able to drive even if you want to. Before surgery, create a list of willing taxi drivers and let them drive your kids to and from basketball or ballet.

- **Babysitting.** This is for you, not your kids. If you don't have a husband who can take off work or a relative who can come stay for a few days, create a schedule prior to surgery and have friends sign up to take shifts staying with you. You don't need to entertain them. You don't even need to be in the same room with them—as long as they can hear your call when you need something. Remember, you might not even be able to get out of a chair without help for a few days.

Resources

1. Beck, Susan, DO. Interview by author. Huxley, Iowa, October 30, 2019.
2. Mayo Clinic Staff. "Lymphedema." MayoClinic.com, December 21, 2017. https://www.mayoclinic.org/diseases-conditions/lymphedema/symptoms-causes/syc-20374682.
3. "When and Where Lymphedema Can Occur." Breastcancer.org, updated August 10, 2016. https://www.breastcancer.org/treatment/lymphedema/when_where.

Chapter 7

I Feel Ugly: Grieving the Loss of Your Breasts and Discovering a New Normal

"Nothing makes a woman more beautiful than the
belief that she is beautiful."
—Sophia Loren

"I think I'm gonna throw up."

Those were the first words that escaped my mouth when I saw my breastless chest for the first time. Technically, I wasn't really breastless since I'd had the first phase of reconstruction the same day as my bilateral mastectomy, but the woman in the mirror looking back at me was disfigured. It was like she'd been mauled by a wild animal who tore at her chest with one giant claw, leaving angry scars where two breasts had been. I felt damaged. I felt ugly.

Corey's reflection also looked back from that mirror. The same mirror he taped a giant piece of paper over a week earlier when I wasn't quite ready to see the new me. Now the paper lay crumpled on the floor and my reflection overwhelmed me. "You don't have to throw up," his reflection in the mirror mouthed to me. "It's okay. You'll be okay. You are beautiful, and it will be okay."

But I wasn't okay, and he held my hair out of my face while I turned around and puked.

They're Just Boobs, Right?

Vomiting was quite unexpected. I was never a big fan of my ultra-small breasts, so I didn't think losing them would have much of an effect on me. When I was first hit with a cancer diagnosis, I put zero thought into how hard it would be to adjust to life without my boobs. I just wanted the cancer out of my body, and if that meant my breasts needed to go too, then that's what I wanted.

But standing in front of the mirror on that cold March morning with Corey, I was struck with the truth of that worn-out phrase, "You don't know what you've got until it's gone." I was indescribably sad that my breasts weren't there anymore. But for goodness' sake, I was alive and cancer-free—certainly I had no reason to be sad, right? Is it even okay to cry over something as superficial as boobs? I constantly fought in my mind against the sadness because I had a funny feeling that being sorrowful about losing my breasts was selfish. My thought life became chaotic and exhausting.

One voice in my head repeatedly hit me with this: *I'm heartbroken that my boobs are gone. I'm not pretty anymore. I don't feel whole. I want to crawl in my bed and cry.* An opposing voice fired back: *They were just boobs. No one died. No one else can even see them. Stop being an idiot and get over it.* These thoughts refused to give my brain a break.

On any given day to the outside world, I'm sure I looked fine. But inside, a battle raged. I felt like I should focus on being thankful the cancer was gone. Thankful that I had the opportunity to spend more years with my husband. Thankful that I would get to watch my boys grow into men. And I *was* thankful for those things. But at the same time, I was extraordinarily sad.

If this is happening to you too, know that you are not alone. Many women who've lost their breasts to cancer have fought the same fight. It's a normal reaction to losing a body part. According to a study in the *British Medical Journal*, the loss of body parts can have overlapping psychological consequences, and though a mastectomy "may have little influence on a woman's functional ability, the effect on her body image will usually be profound."[1]

This principle held true with survivor Ronell, who was just as surprised as I was by the way the loss of her breasts affected her. She was recovering from a nipple-sparing bilateral mastectomy with immediate reconstruction when the sadness hit. Aside from her scars, she said her new breasts looked perky and youthful, but the loss still felt profound.

"It was very awkward to wake up [from surgery] fit with this set of twenty-year-old breasts when I was forty-four. I wasn't ready for that. I kind of hated the whole thing," she said. "I avoided mirrors. Avoided changing in front of my husband. I avoided a lot of stuff for a while."

Once her body began to physically heal, she still fought a mental and emotional battle. The first time she tried on a swimsuit, she cried. "I put it on and just cried. And they looked good. That's the thing. They looked good. But I hated them because they were different."

Ronell's breasts didn't even look ugly to her like mine did to me, and the loss was still hard to deal with. She kept wishing she could get past it. "I knew enough about the stages of grief to recognize that's what I was doing, but that didn't make it better."

April Stearns, founder and editor of *Wildfire Magazine*, had a unilateral mastectomy and chose to go flat. Like me, when she was in the decision-making phase, she only wanted the cancer out of her body and gave very little thought to the body she would be left with. But while watching television with her husband one evening, she was struck by the cleavage of one of the female characters and wondered if she'd made the right decision.

"I looked down at my chest. I had no cleavage anymore. No symmetry. No youth or vitality anymore, it seemed. Just one breast on one side that now looked a bit sad to me on its own, and a six-inch scar on the other side. Up till that moment I hadn't given much thought to how my new chest would look. I was concerned with simply getting the tumor out of my body and getting on with life. Now I realized that 'getting on with life' would also mean coming to terms with living in a body I no longer recognized as my own."[2]

And that is a struggle for many women when cancer takes their breasts. How do we learn to live well in these bodies we no longer recognize as our own?

The Value of Our Bodies

Is it okay to be sad my boobs are gone? Can I grieve a missing piece of my body? I wrestled with these questions for a long while. And I ended up looking outside of myself to come to a conclusion. Culture, the natural world around me, and the Bible all helped shape my perspective.

Our culture definitely values the feminine form. From advertisements to television shows to social media, you'd have to walk around with your eyes closed to not see that physical beauty is idolized in our great nation. Culture screams at us that physical beauty is the end goal. Perfection is the objective, and I am not immune to striving for it. In fact, I color my hair every four weeks to hide my premature gray. (Seriously, by age forty I didn't have much of my natural color left. My mom found my first gray hair at one of my high school track meets. I was seventeen.) I'm self-conscious of the unibrow that I work hard to keep under control with my handy-dandy tweezers. And I'm a little embarrassed every time I wear flip-flops because I'm missing a toenail. I want to look good, and I'm easily embarrassed by my deficiencies. I believe the influence of culture is partially to blame.

But one thing I know about culture is that it lies—a lot. We are shaped by the advertising fed to us by corporations and businesses. Their goal is not our self-esteem. Their goal is to sell their products, and one way they do this is by manipulating us to become dissatisfied with ourselves. So did the fact that I was heartbroken about my boobs mean that I had taken the cultural bait yet again? That I had fallen for the claim that better cleavage equals a better life? Maybe that's a piece of it. But there's more to it than that.

The natural world, unlike our culture, speaks the truth of physical beauty without saying a word and without anything to sell. The mountains don't lie. There is a reason over three million people visit Rocky Mountain National Park each year. The ocean waves don't lie. Resort after resort lines the world's most gorgeous beaches because people are drawn to the beauty. Even the rows of golden Iowa corn speak truth in silence: awe-inspiring perfectly straight rows line up for miles along Midwestern roads. And right now, at this moment, I am typing these words in a tiny cabin in the woods, surrounded by plant life, singing birds, and a creek that is flowing strong from heavy spring rains. It's a writer's dream, and it's beautiful.

In silence, all these things speak loudly the truth that there is beauty in physical things. And if the things we find in nature are breathtakingly beautiful, then certainly the human form can be considered beautiful as well. Undoubtedly, my breasts that are no longer there held their own real beauty. As author and artist Jess C. Scott puts it, "The human body is the best work of art."

Because my faith is key to who I am, I added another piece to this beauty equation—intelligent design. Whether you believe in the God of the Bible, or simply in the existence of an intelligent designer, it's fitting to wrestle with the question of whether or not a higher power would create something as detailed and purposeful as the human body and not place value on its design. The Bible focuses much on inner beauty and character, but some key places speak of external beauty too.

"May her breasts satisfy you always," King Solomon writes in the Proverbs (Proverbs 5:19 [NIV]). If my breasts were supposed to satisfy Corey always, surely they were valuable. The tiny book of Esther tucked into the Old Testament also speaks of physical beauty. Esther was the beautiful maiden chosen to be the queen of Persia. And though her internal beauty far outweighed her external beauty, her outward appearance was a stepping stone on the path that gave her the opportunity to save the Jewish nation from massacre. Song of Solomon is a sensual book filled with references to physical beauty. If you are up for an interesting read, take a few minutes and check out the super weird imagery written about physical beauty. I can only assume that when it was written, having your breasts compared to a species of antelope (Song of Solomon 4:5 [NIV]) was a compliment. These sections of the Bible increased my assurance that physical beauty has value.

I believe God is an artist and that He created beauty. He placed it in the mountains, the ocean waves, the rows of golden Iowa corn. And He placed it in you and me, and that includes our breasts.

The Value of Our Spirit

On the flip side, it's important to recognize our inner beauty in this process—the value of our spirit. Though culture tells us differently, internal beauty is vastly more important than external. And as with external beauty, we can see evidence if we take a step back and look outside of ourselves.

Some of the most revered characters in history were not physically beautiful. But because they did things that were beautiful, we think of the beauty of their character and their inner spirit. The things we see become less, and the things we can't see become more. Google a photo of Abraham Lincoln. He was an ugly dude. But we don't remember him for his physical body. We remember him for leading the nation in the abolition of slavery. And I'm told Beethoven was ugly as well. One article describes him as a short, ugly man who was generally unkempt with a pockmarked face.[3] I've only seen pencil drawings of him, so I don't know how accurate the description is, but when I think of the nineteenth-century composer, I don't think of an ugly man. I think about beautiful music. And through his music, he becomes beautiful. When unattractive people do beautiful things, those people somehow become more beautiful in our eyes.

And it's not just famous historical people. Think of your favorite "real life" people. The ones you enjoy being around. The ones you respect. The ones you desire to emulate. Do you find them physically attractive? They're probably not supermodels by the world's standards, but I'm guessing when you look at them you see beauty. The thing is, when a person is beautiful on the inside, it shines through on the outside. We can't look at that friend or relative or mentor and see an average-looking person. What we see instead is beauty.

My aunt Marilyn radiates this kind of beauty. If you passed her on the street, you would probably see a regular-looking woman. But when I look at her, I see beauty. I can't look at her and see only her hair, mouth, and eyes. I see a woman whose parents died in a car accident when she was sixteen years old, leaving her and her eighteen-year-old sister to raise their younger siblings. I see a woman who lost a husband at a young age to autoimmune hepatitis of the liver and, later, almost a son to the same disease. I see the strength, joy, faith, and humility with which she has overcome these things, and I can't help but think of her as one of the most beautiful people I know. The beauty of the spirit within affects the way we see the beauty on the outside.

Even if you aren't a Bible reader, there's a fair chance you've heard of the *Proverbs 31 woman*. She is the picture of perfection. Much is commended on her wisdom, compassion, business skills, and ability to provide for her family. All things of internal value. The only verse in that whole chapter that mentions external beauty describes it as "fleeting" (Proverbs 31:30 [NIV]). Physical beauty exists, but it is fleeting. The way that verse is tucked into that particular chapter provides a good perspective check for me when weighing the value of external and internal beauty.

Regardless of your view of the Bible, having a balanced view is an important part of the healing process. Do yourself a favor and recognize that the boobs you were born with had beauty and value but also that your reconstructed or flat chest carries beauty and value of its own. And don't forget to weigh your spirit more heavily than your body. If we can keep an appropriate amount of tension between the two, we can start making our way to a healthy body image.

Grieving Our Boobs

It's impossible for us to grieve the piece that is missing if we don't allow ourselves to believe that piece carried value. The point at which we allow ourselves to believe there is a certain amount of value to our physical appearance is the point at which grieving our breasts can start. If we convince ourselves that our physical bodies should be ignored, we layer guilt on top of heartache when the sadness creeps in. When we don't believe we have the right to feel sad, we don't give ourselves room to grieve. And I believe grieving our breasts is not only healthy, but—for a lot of us—necessary.

But even when we get to the point that we can say, "Yes, my boobs were valuable," we still have another hurdle to cross, and that is the fact that death does not play a role in this grief. We grow up associating grief with death. We believe that grieving is something we do when someone we love, or maybe a pet, dies. It's expected, it's immediate, and it's usually life altering. It is not something we do after the wonders of modern medicine remove cancerous breasts from our bodies, even if they were beautiful. At least, that's what I thought.

Then I read this book called *Wednesdays Were Pretty Normal* by Michael Kelley. The book about the author's walk through leukemia with his little boy is what ultimately convinced me that it was okay to grieve my lost boobs. Kelley says, "We often think about the grieving process exclusively in terms of people. You lose someone close to you, and you lament that loss in personal and profound ways. But the same process happens, I believe, to other areas of life too. . . . In the end, grieving is about loss and finding your way through life without the thing that's not there anymore."[4]

Let me repeat that: *grieving is about loss and finding your way through life without the thing that's not there anymore.* That idea was profound to me. My boobs had been with me for forty years when the surgeon took them away. They caused me angst in my late elementary school years when all of my friends had bras and I didn't. They grew to almost fill out an A cup bikini when I was in high school. They filled with milk, not one time, but for three separate seasons of breastfeeding baby boys. They provided sexual stimulation. They made me look and feel feminine. And they were gone. And I was trying to find my way through life without them.

Michael Kelley has no idea that he gave me permission to grieve my breasts. (Maybe that's good, because it would probably weird him out a little.) But what a relief it was the day I could say, "Yes, it's okay that I miss my breasts. It's okay to cry. It's okay to grieve."

Another survivor, Ronell, had a similar experience with grieving for her breasts too. She remembers feelings of anger as she walked through her grief. "I was mad for a while. . . . I struggled in the summer when I had to put on a swimsuit. Trying one on triggered the tears and frustration." More than a year after surgery, Ronell still struggles with the scars, but she is growing more comfortable with her new boobs.

It took time for another survivor to come to terms with the *new her* too. But after seven years, April finally came to a place of feeling at home in her new body. "I still find cleavage enviable, and I wish I could wear shirts and dresses that reveal it, but I no longer wonder if I made a mistake in choosing against reconstruction."

The How-To of Grieving

Speaking about grieving the loss of a body part still feels weird to me sometimes, but I did indeed grieve the loss of my breasts, and I did have to train my brain to believe I could be a beautiful woman with fake, scarred, numb, nipple-less boobs. In reality, the grief still creeps in sometimes, but I now feel *normal* in my grief. Like it's just another piece of the healing process that comes after cancer enters your world.

If you are struggling the way Ronell, April, and I struggled, I hope that this chapter plays a role in your grieving process and that my words can do for you what Michael Kelley's words did for me. I'd love to be able to give you a step-by-step guide to walk through your grief, but I can't. Looking back, I can't even fully decipher whether or not I made my way through each of the five stages of grief we all learned about in Psych 101. But I can tell you about the key things I did to get myself from one side of grief to the other.

I Fought the Voices

It started with fighting the voices in my head. First was the voice who told me I was ugly and not whole. The next one told me I didn't have the right to grieve. The voices didn't turn themselves off because I had an "aha" moment reading a book about childhood cancer, but I did start recognizing the lies and calling them out. We all have regular running conversations in our head, and it's easy to let the voices keep on talking and give ourselves over to them. But I wanted my mind to be in a healthy place, so I fought.

Fighting voices in our head sounds kind of loopy, and *it's not easy, but it's necessary.* Vincent van Gogh is credited with saying, "If you hear a voice within you say you cannot paint, then by all means paint and that voice will be silenced."[5] Fighting the voices in our head is not a new concept, and it requires action on our part.

According to an article in *Psychology Today*, we all experience negative voices in our head. These voices are "automatic, fear-based rules for living that act like inner bullies, keeping us stuck in the same old cycles and hampering our spontaneous enjoyment of life and our ability to live and love freely." The article encourages the acknowledgment of and empathetic connecting with unresolved fears and unmet needs to become more mentally flexible and free.[6]

In the New Testament of the Bible, a section states the same thing from a faith-based perspective. It says we must demolish arguments (in our heads) that set themselves up against the knowledge of God, and we must take our thoughts captive, making them obedient to Christ (2 Corinthians 10:5 [NIV]).

Each of these examples requires us to become active participants to fight the voices, but it's impossible to passively go from wrong to right thinking. It takes mental effort. Here's a couple of examples of the conversations that took place in my head:

Lying voice: "You are ugly. Your natural boobs are gone forever, and these fake ones will always be ugly."

Voice of truth: "I am beautiful. My boobs are different, but they are beautiful in their own way."

Lying voice: "You are being ridiculous. Stop crying. They were just boobs. Get over it."

Voice of truth: "I am not ridiculous. They were not *just* boobs. They were a piece of me that I will never get back. It's okay to be sad. It's okay to grieve."

This is not a one-time fight. Like most of life's struggles, it takes daily battles to win the war. But it's so worth the effort.

I Found an Outlet

Recognize the way you deal with grief and give yourself the resources to do it well. That may mean buying a punching bag, joining a weight-training program, writing in a journal, meeting with a counselor, or any combination of those things. Just be sure to find something that helps you move forward.

I'm a writer, so I wrote. A lot. Journaling has always helped me make sense of the things going on in my head. But you know what else I did? I grabbed my magic blanket (see Chapter 1) and a pillow and I lay down by myself in front of my fireplace and cried and cried and cried.

I considered visiting a counselor, but I never took that step. Because I had such a good relationship with Corey and a tight-knit network of friends, I received a form of therapy from the people in my life every day. But there's great value in walking through this with the help of a trained professional too, and you are in good company if you choose to do so.

I Believed My Loved Ones

This one might seem like a no-brainer, but sometimes I let myself think that the people I love just say things because they have to, not necessarily because they believe they're true.

Corey often tells me I'm more beautiful today than I was two decades ago when we got married. When I look in the mirror, I have a hard time seeing that, and I could easily choose not to believe him. I could also choose not to believe him when he tells me he still thinks my body is beautiful, even though it's missing one of his favorite parts. But one thing I know for sure is that I didn't marry a liar. If I ever start to question his claims, I need only to remind myself that Corey is the most humble, honest, and kind person I know. If he says I'm beautiful, then dang it, I am beautiful. And if your spouse or significant other tells you that you are beautiful, *believe it.* You are beautiful.

Cry the tears. Grieve the loss. Fight the lying voices. Listen to your loved ones. And tell yourself you are beautiful until you believe it.

Resources

1. Maguire, Peter, and Parkes, Colin Murray. 1998. "Surgery and Loss of Body Parts." *BMJ* 316, no. 7137: 1086–88. https://www.ncbi.nlm.nih.gov/pmc/articles/PMC1112908/.

2. Stearns, April. *Wildfire Magazine* Newsletter, June 1, 2019.

3. Heider, Hildburg, and Berg, Marita. "Glimpses of Beethoven in Society and with Friends." DW.com, September 9, 2011. https://www.dw.com/en/glimpses-of-beethoven-in-society-and-with-friends/a-6614678.

4. Kelley, Michael. *Wednesdays Were Pretty Normal: A Boy, Cancer and God.* Nashville, TN: B&H Publishing Group, 2012.

5. Johnson, Patrick. "If You Hear a Voice Within You Say You Cannot Paint." *Beyond Quarter Life*, October 13, 2014. https://beyondquarterlife.com/hear-voice-within-say-paint/.

6. Greenberg, Melanie. "When the Voice Inside Your Head Turns Bad." *Psychology Today*, April 18, 2012. https://www.psychologytoday.com/us/blog/the-mindful-self-express/201204/when-the-voice-inside-your-head-turns-bad.

Chapter 8

Sex with New Boobs: Reconstruction Is a Game Changer

"It is an absolute human certainty that no one can know his own beauty or perceive a sense of his own worth until it has been reflected back to him in the mirror of another loving, caring human being."
—John Joseph Powell, *The Secret of Staying in Love*

Sometimes I get mad at God. I don't want to, but I do. I don't get mad about the cancer. I wasn't happy about it by any means, but for some weird reason it felt like we were due for some rough waters when I was diagnosed. In our seventeen years of marriage leading up to breast cancer, the only major loss we faced was a miscarriage. I don't want to diminish the pain of that experience, because it hurt. A lot. But God blessed us with three amazing, healthy boys, and if a miscarriage was the only really hard thing I had to face in nearly two decades of life, I consider that pretty smooth sailing.

My frustration toward God was about sex. How awful is that? Sex is supposed to be this wonderful, beautiful connection of mind, spirit, and body. A God-given gift. But now my body was broken, and sex wasn't wonderful or beautiful. It was hard. My newly created breasts were like foreign objects to me. Ugly, distracting, foreign objects. It literally took us years of marriage to figure out the whole sex thing, and once we finally got to a satisfying spot, it was like God said, "Okay, now let's see how you do without boobs."

It felt so unfair.

Ninety percent of the time, living without my natural breasts is relatively easy. I have days I hardly even think about it. But when I am naked with my husband, it's impossible to avoid the reality of my reconstructed breasts. Maybe sex without boobs hasn't affected you like it has me. I know women are aroused in different ways, and for some, breasts may play a minimal role in the sexual experience. I hope that's the case for you. I hope that in the midst of all the hard things that cancer brings, this is one thing that is not a struggle in your life. But if it is, know that I am right there with you. My breasts, specifically my nipples, played a major role for me in sex. Unfortunately, my breasts are now nearly numb and I don't even have nipples. The key piece of me that used to get my body moving in the direction of sexual satisfaction is gone forever. And sometimes that makes me a little mad.

It's not that sex is bad now or that I've lost the ability to reach a climax. It's just considerably harder. Because of that, sometimes I don't want to make the effort. If you can't relate, think of it this way. Imagine your favorite café is down the road several miles, and for years you've driven your car there a few times a week to enjoy some coffee and a muffin. Then one day someone steals your car and you are left with only a bicycle. You can still get to the café on your bike, but it takes a lot more time and energy. Some days, you just don't feel up to all of the pedaling. That's what sex is like for me. It can be really good, but some days I can't muster up the energy to *hop on the bike and head to the coffee shop.* At those times, I end up frustrated with myself and feel as if I'm failing my husband. Ugh.

I had the opportunity to interview psychologist and physical intimacy expert Dr. Juli Slattery of Authentic Intimacy, and she provided reassurance that this struggle is normal, even for couples without breast cancer as part of their story. Add mastectomy and breast reconstruction to the equation, and the struggle is amplified. Slattery said the best advice she can give couples struggling after breast cancer alters their sex life is to change their mindset on the obstacles. "Instead of viewing [reconstructed breasts] as killing your sex life, begin to view them as a team challenge. Your greatest obstacles can actually become the most powerful invitations to true intimacy," she said. "You don't have to learn to listen, forgive, and sacrifice when sex is easy. Those things are forged through the disappointments and conflicts."[1]

I know and believe this, but I still struggle. I don't necessarily want to learn to listen, forgive, and sacrifice in the midst of this. I just want to have good sex. Sex like we used to have. So I start to question God. *Why? Why did you do this to me?* And then I wonder why I did this to myself. The big "What if?" comes into play. What if I had kept my right breast? The removal of the left was by necessity, but the right was by choice. A choice I made so I wouldn't live my life wondering if cancer would come back in the other breast. But what if I had kept my healthy boob? Would living with the worry of recurrence have been better than living with the loss of both breasts? Probably not. But that doesn't keep the decision from haunting me sometimes when I long for the intimacy Corey and I had before cancer.

When I look back objectively, though, I can see that a bilateral mastectomy is the decision God led me to, and I don't regret making it. As I wrestled with whether or not to have my non-cancerous breast removed, not one person I sought counsel from encouraged me to keep my cancer-free breast. In fact, one woman who opted for a single mastectomy told me that in hindsight she wished she would've had both breasts removed. And another initially had a single mastectomy and went back to have the other breast removed a few years later to ease her worry. All signs pointed to me having both breasts removed. So that's what I did.

The what-ifs are useless. When we start going down that road, we need to remind ourselves that there's no going back—only forward. I am confident that Corey and I will get back to where we were with intimacy before cancer. In fact, we've made strides in the past couple years. And because we know everything good is worth striving for, we will continue the work of developing our intimate relationship.

Initial Return to Intimacy

I can give you no formula to use for your initial return to sexual intimacy. Just like no two marriages are alike, no two roads to sexual intimacy after mastectomy and breast reconstruction are exactly the same. For some, it will be easier than others. But know that many couples find sex at this time in their lives a difficult challenge, and at the very least, there will be a learning curve.

In the days and often weeks after surgery, sex is not even possible. When you can't lift your arms over your head to dress yourself, the thought of being intimate is off the radar. But as healing begins, so can the process of returning to intimacy.

Your doctor may advise you on how long to wait after surgery for sex, or he or she may tell you to take it at your own pace and return to intimacy when you feel ready. But what should it look like? How should you start? How do you return to this important part of your relationship when cancer changed what you knew?

I hesitate to write this because it's slightly mortifying to think of the possibility of my teenage boys reading it, but oral sex might be a good place to start. It isn't for everyone, but it is a gentler way to return to intimacy. It's easier to avoid contact with the tender places still healing on your body while participating in oral sex, so it can be a good early option to provide satisfaction to one or both of you.

Another thing to consider when you return to "regular" sex is body position. According to Marc Silver's book *Breast Cancer Husband*, Dr. Megan Mills, director of psychosocial oncology at Chicago's Rush Cancer Institute, said the wife may prefer to be on top, because on top she can decide how active to be and how far to go. She is in control and the husband "doesn't have to worry about when it's too much."[2]

This was the case for us. I was on top and we took it very slow. Corey was patient with me and didn't push at all. Not only was I on top, but before we made that first attempt, we purposely kept our expectations low. Primarily, this meant me offering myself to Corey with zero expectation of an orgasm for myself and Corey not allowing himself to feel disappointed that he couldn't yet satisfy me sexually.

I knew that I wanted to be intimate with him, but I also knew that I wasn't ready for the whole shebang. Adjusting expectations actually took a ton of pressure off of me. Knowing he wasn't expecting to *satisfy* me released him from the pressure of performing. And I found deep joy in knowing that I was loving my husband in a way he needed to be loved. Going from being nearly completely helpless (needing help getting dressed and even getting off the toilet) to being able to do this little thing for him physically made me feel good.

Dr. Slattery says, "Your sexual relationship isn't about how often you have sex or how great the sex is; it's about being on a journey with your spouse."[3] Oh, what a journey it becomes after you've had your breasts removed!

Others' experiences are similar to mine. Bothered and distracted by the lack of feeling in her new breasts, intimacy was hard and upset Ronell. But she knew that even though it was hard, it was something she wanted and needed to work through. "I think it's important not to withhold intimacy out of fear. I just needed to understand that and take it slow," which she and her husband did. They are now a few years past surgery and have found it worth the effort, as they now have a healthy intimate relationship.

But as I stated earlier, some women have an easier time getting back into the groove. This was true for Angelia, who returned to intimacy just one week after her bilateral mastectomy with direct-to-implant reconstruction. She found that the change created some positives for her sex life. "Both nipples were spared and my breasts are actually larger now, which adds to the excitement." The fact that one of her breasts actually regained sensation later on after a follow-up surgery has also allowed her and her husband to have a satisfying sexual relationship post-mastectomy and reconstruction.

Psychological and Emotional Obstacles

Not just the obvious physical change affects sex after mastectomy—you must wade through emotional and psychological changes as well. My boobs played a huge role in sex. Now they were gone. And the reason they were gone was cancer. In the early days, intimacy always reminded me of the cancer. I could generally go about my day without cancer at the forefront of my mind, but during intimacy it was a different story. It's really challenging to get your mind in the right place for sex when the act itself makes you think about a disease that takes people's lives. And it's not a cakewalk for our husbands either.

Corey wanted to please me, but he was afraid of hurting me physically, and he was really sad himself that my breasts were gone. He had to concentrate on being physically gentle while trying to hide his sadness. He carried around guilt over the sadness because he felt being sad was selfish. He wanted to be thankful that his wife was cancer-free, but he couldn't keep the sadness at bay. The truth is we were both sad about the loss of my boobs, and we both needed to grieve. And part of working through that grieving meant committing to intimacy, even if it was hard.

More than once our attempts at intimacy were halted by tears.

Sometimes his. Sometimes mine. We came to know that this was a possibility we always needed to prepare for. We definitely grieved the loss of what we had in the past, but we didn't quit trying to accept and even embrace our new reality. We knew that we wanted a healthy marriage, and having a healthy marriage includes a healthy sex life. So when the tears came and disrupted the intimate moment, we rested in the fact that we were both committed to see this through, that this was only a little hiccup in the process. We loved each other deeply, and knowing that helped with the healing.

Survivor Angelia and her husband, Dan, had a different experience. They found sex actually aided the healing instead of being something that needed healing itself.

"The night before surgery, I was a mess. . . . Right up to the moment of surgery, I could hardly speak or breathe without crying. After surgery and after I was off the strong pain meds, we needed to feel close to each other. [Our first sexual experience after surgery] wasn't physical at all; it was an emotional and spiritual connection that we needed to help us recover from the craziness we had just been through. We actually found this life-changing event brought us to a much more intimate place."

Maybe you can relate to my story, maybe your experience is closer to Angelia's, or maybe you find yourself somewhere in between. But wherever you land on the spectrum, know that you are not alone. And be encouraged that the struggle it takes to get to a good place is worth the time and effort.

Body Image and Intimacy

Body image is a huge obstacle psychologically for women as they return to intimacy. I explored body image in Chapter 7, but I think it's necessary to touch on in this chapter as well, because when do we think more about our body image than when we are naked?

The world spews images of attractive, sexy women at us every day from a thousand different angles. We, unfortunately, live in a culture where all physical flaws are photoshopped into oblivion and we are left with images impressed on our minds that simply aren't true—images that cause us to think less of ourselves because we know we can never attain that perfection. When we've lost our breasts, there's another level added to the body image struggle, and it can be a challenge to feel sexy.

But Dr. Slattery says that we, as women (regardless of whether we have our natural breasts or not), will benefit from changing our mindset about the word "sexy." She recommends thinking of sexiness as less of a look and more of an attitude. "You have to 'learn' to become sexy. It's not something that just happens. In fact, you may need to relearn being sexy as you transition into different stages of marriage and confront new challenges."[4] For many women, those stages may include new wrinkles, added weight, skin spots, or graying and thinning hair. For us, the immediate challenge is the change to our chests.

In those first few months of post-cancer sex, not only did I not strive to reach a climax, but I also wore a tank top. It may sound counterproductive to ignore this new piece of me that I will spend the rest of my life with, but I had to take one step at a time. I found that if I kept my chest covered, I thought about my boobs less and focused on Corey more, and I could more easily feel sexy and become aroused myself.

When I became more comfortable with this new sexual experience and my new body, I left the shirt behind. The shirt trick was a little thing, but it proved extremely helpful to me. So go ahead and wear a shirt for a while if you need to. Experts recommend the cover-up method as well. As quoted in *Breast Cancer Husband*, Dr. Mills suggests sexy, short lingerie and dim, almost dark, lighting to take the focus off the breasts.[5]

The goal is not to have great sex from the start but to work toward a place where both you and your husband are emotionally and physically satisfied. If you find the journey frustrating at times, remember that most valuable things we achieve in life take significant commitment and effort.

In Dr. Slattery's decades of experience, she has found that the body image issue is much more of a struggle for us as women than it is for our men.[6] If you are nervous about whether or not your husband finds you less attractive with your reconstructed breasts, it's likely he doesn't struggle the same way you do. Like Corey, he may feel some sadness and it may take him some time to get used to the new you, but he will likely still see right past your scars to his beautiful bride.

"While most men appreciate the work we do to look healthy, fit, and attractive, they are even more appreciative of the energy we put into the mental state of sexiness," Slattery said. "Men are naturally enticed by invitation." If this is true, using our words, our clothing, and our environment to invite our husbands to intimacy with us is more valuable than looking like the model on the front cover of *Vogue*. (We all know she doesn't really exist anyway.)

Hormone Therapy and Intimacy

According to WebMD, about 80 percent of all breast cancer tumors are estrogen-receptor positive, which means the cancer feeds on estrogen.[7] Women with these types of tumors are generally prescribed an estrogen-blocking drug for five to ten years after treatment. Pre-menopausal women normally take a drug called tamoxifen, and post-menopausal women are prescribed aromatase inhibitors. Maybe you are currently taking or will be taking one of these drugs in the future.

The super awesome thing about these drugs is that they reduce the probability of breast cancer recurrence by 50 percent, according to Dr. Robert Wesolowski, assistant professor at the Ohio State University Comprehensive Cancer Center.[8] The not-so-good news is they can have an effect on libido. Both types of drugs come with the possibility of a variety of side effects that I won't go into in this chapter, but one of the most common is a decreased appetite for sex. Aromatase inhibitors also come with a high likelihood of vaginal dryness, which further adds to sexual complications.

I wish I could tell you there is a magic pill you can take to make it all better, but there's not. A couple of FDA-approved medicines help women with a low libido, but they are not a fix-it-all solution.

Flibanserin is a central nervous system drug that works to decrease inhibition while increasing excitation. It comes in the form of a pill that you take every evening, but it's cost prohibitive for many women (a one-month prescription is approximately $800). It is also recommended that alcohol not be consumed within two hours of taking the pill because the combination increases the risk of orthostatic hypertension.

Bremelanotide is a shot you give yourself in the belly or thigh before having sex. It's also a central nervous system drug and works a lot like Viagra. Doctors recommend no more than eight shots a month. This option is also cost prohibitive for some (it is around $100 for four shots).

Recently a new, non-prescription option has become available. An l-arginine supplement (Ristela) is available online through Bonafide, a company that focuses on creating non-prescription solutions for women's health issues. According to Susan Beck, DO, the benefits of this option are threefold—increased desire, arousal, and climax.[9] But it must be taken daily for about three months in order to build up in the system and be effective. The cost of this option (at about $150 for three months) is significantly less than the two prescriptions currently available.

If you are considering any of these options, speak with your oncologist. It may also be beneficial to speak with a member of the North American Menopause Society (NAMS). The nonprofit organization's expertise involves walking with women going through issues brought on by menopause, and many of the sexual side effects women undergo in breast cancer treatment are similar to menopausal symptoms.

Personal lubricants are another option to aid in the return to a healthy sex life. Replens is a popular over-the-counter vaginal moisturizer insert that should be used regularly to achieve the greatest benefit, not just in association with sex. (Prescription vaginal moisturizer inserts, including Imvexxy and Intrarosa, are also available.) You can also purchase a wide variety of external lubricants used during sex at drugstores and online. Dr. Leslie Schover, professor of behavioral science in the cancer prevention division at the University of Texas MD Anderson Cancer Center, recommends using water-based or silicone-based vaginal lubricants in addition to using a vaginal moisturizer (like Replens) regularly. But when this isn't enough, she says a local vaginal estrogen is the next least risky option.[10]

Estrogen-containing vaginal creams are considered somewhat controversial, but medical professionals like Dr. Schover and gynecologist Melanie Bone recommend them for women who are struggling. Bone says that because very little of an already-low dose of estrogen in the creams absorbs systemically, they don't pose a risk to the user.[11] Susan Beck agrees, and adds that women on hormone therapy (tamoxifen or an aromatase inhibitor) actually have a hedge of protection from the estrogen. She recommends informing your doctor if you plan to keep using estrogen-containing vaginal creams after going off of hormone therapy.

Yet another option to consider to help improve your sex life after breast cancer is something called MonaLisa Touch. This is a painless, non-surgical laser procedure that stimulates the production of collagen on the vaginal mucosa.[12]

Thankfully, not all women struggle with loss of libido from hormone blockers. I've been on tamoxifen since 2016 and have noticed very little side effects. I consider this a great blessing, as I have struggled with sex for other cancer-related reasons.

Preparation Is Invaluable

Maybe you are just starting this journey. Maybe you are still making decisions about surgical options. Maybe you are so overwhelmed with the thought of cancer that sex is far, far from your mind. That's okay. You need to walk through each piece of this journey as it comes. But being aware that sex may become a hurdle down the road will allow your mind a chance to better prepare for it in advance.

It's been several years since my reconstruction was completed, and Corey and I are in a pretty good place. We're not in a perfect place, but we keep moving forward and are more in love now than ever before. Our biggest issue with sex now isn't even my changed body but the fact that we have high school–age children who always seem to be awake. Can I get an "Amen" from those of you with teens in the house?

Sex Suggestions from Psychologist Dr. Juli Slattery

- Schedule sex. A lot of the energy is mental. Having time to get your mind in gear can make a big difference.
- Tell your husband what he can do to get you in the mood. A back rub? Putting the kids to bed? A specific way he talks to you to get your mind into it?
- Be open to your body responding when you don't think it will. A lot of times a woman will have zero desire, but once she begins with foreplay, she finds herself somewhat receptive. Don't be stubborn with the mindset of "I just can't get there."
- Initiate when you are ready. Couples might get into a cycle where the man always initiates and the wife is in a position of always saying no. It's important to break this pattern. Determine that you will initiate sex once this week. Look for that opportunity when you have the brain space and energy for intimacy.

Suggestions from Couples Who've Been There

- Splurge on a night in a hotel prior to surgery and focus on enjoying each other—a kind of farewell to your breasts.
- Wear a tank top, a T-shirt, or breast-covering lingerie when you resume sex if you find yourself distracted by your chest.
- Lower your sexual expectations. Don't expect to climax right out of the chute.
- Communicate. Talk to each other about body image, how you feel physically, and what does and doesn't work for you in your new post-mastectomy intimacy world.
- Try the sensate focus technique.[13] (You can find a link to instructions in the resource section at the end of this chapter.)
- Find a trusted friend who is not your spouse who you feel comfortable talking and processing through the sexual challenges with. Sometimes it helps to have a sounding board who is not involved.
- Be patient.
- If funds allow, plan a trip after you have healed and found yourselves a new normal. Extended alone time to focus on each other can be exceptionally healing.

Resources

1. Slattery, Juli. Email message to author. Iowa, September 30, 2019.
2. Silver, Marc. *Breast Cancer Husband: How to Help Your Wife (and Yourself) During Diagnosis, Treatment and Beyond.* Emmaus, PA: Rodale Books, 2004. 174.
3. Slattery, Juli. email message to author.
4. Ibid.
5. Silver, Marc. *Breast Cancer Husband.*
6. Slattery, Juli. email message to author.
7. "What is Hormone Receptor-Positive Breast Cancer?" WebMD.com, updated July 1, 2020. https://www.webmd.com/breast-cancer/qa/what-is-hormone-receptorpositive-breast-cancer.
8. Pietrangelo, Ann. "Tamoxifen Helps Prevent Breast Cancer, But Women Are Still Reluctant to Take It." Healthline, December 10, 2018. https://www.healthline.com/health-news/why-women-are-reluctant-to-take-tamoxifen-to-prevent-breast-cancer.
9. Beck, Susan, DO. Interview by author. Iowa, December 15, 2019.
10. "Staying Sexual: Cancer and Intimacy." Everyday Health, updated February 5, 2008. https://www.everydayhealth.com/cancer/webcasts/staying-sexual-cancer-and-intimacy.aspx.
11. Boyles, Salynn. "Sex Complaints Common after Breast Cancer." WebMD. com, September 23, 2010. https://www.webmd.com/breast-cancer/news/20100923/sex-complaints-common-after-breast-cancer#1.
12. "The New Laser Therapy for the Prevention and Care of Your Vaginal Health." MonaLisa Touch, accessed December 16, 2019. https://www.monalisatouch.com/monalisatouch-the-laser-therapy/.
13. "Sensate Focus." Cornell Health, October 18, 2019. https://health.cornell.edu/sites/health/files/pdf-library/sensate-focus.pdf.

Chapter 9
This Is Hard for Him Too: A Husband's Perspective

"Marriage is an attempt to solve problems together
that you didn't even have when you were on your own."
—Eddie Cantor

A photo hangs in our house of Corey standing at the top of the world, arms outstretched, and a big smile on his face. The sign he's standing beside reads *Mount Kilimanjaro—Congratulations—You are now at Uhuru Peak, Tanzania, 19,341 ft.* It was taken in August of 2017. A year and a half after I was diagnosed with breast cancer. I love that picture.

I tend to be a pretty frugal person, and a hike to the top of Africa's tallest mountain is not an inexpensive endeavor. But I believe it was worth every penny. I also believe that, in a way, it was a gift. Though Corey enjoys climbing mountains in the United States, he never would've sought out a trip this indulgent on his own. But it presented itself to him at the right moment.

Multiple times as he considered the trip, he said, "I shouldn't go. It's too much money." But I pushed him toward it. He took amazing care of me during my cancer year, giving up a lot for my sake, and I thought a couple weeks climbing a mountain with some buddies might give him a chance to unwind and process what we'd just gone through together. That mountain climbing money could have become a new kitchen, but the picture of my man on top of that mountain is infinitely more valuable than stainless steel appliances and granite countertops.

Your husband probably didn't climb Mount Kilimanjaro after you reached the other side of treatment. (You may not even have a husband or a significant other, in which case you can skip ahead to the next chapter.) But chances are your man needs or needed some way to decompress after it was over. Though the cancer is oh-so-hard on us, the women whose bodies it invaded, it also takes a toll on the men who love us.

Fix It

The afternoon I received my diagnosis, I remember Corey crying and saying, "I wish I could take this for you. Why can't it be me instead?" It's heart-wrenching for our husbands to watch us go through painful things. For a lot of guys, there's a feeling of utter helplessness. And because most guys are wired to fix things, being helpless is a very tough spot for them. As protectors and comforters, our men long to take our pain away. But cancer and the physical and emotional pain it causes is something they can't fix. So if your husband behaves in a way that is frustrating to you, it might be because he isn't sure how to handle a problem he can't fix.

Studies show that male brains are often wired to be "emotional fixers" in relationships. In an article at Today.com, author of *The Male Brain* and neuropsychiatrist Dr. Louann Brizendine explores differences between male and female brains that help explain why some men act the way they do. She says, "It's very much men wanting to fix it when he's feeling an uncomfortable emotion. So these things can really cause conflicts in relationships because she feels not heard by him and thinks he's just running over her."[1]

Because he is wired to fix things, your man's support might rub you the wrong way sometimes. But chances are he's in no way trying to hurt you; he's simply working through this diagnosis the best way he knows how. In his book *Breast Cancer Husband*, Marc Silver says, "Our wives want to tell us how they're feeling; we may feel uncomfortable listening. Part of the reason may be our male desire to fix things. And how do you fix a bad feeling? By making it go away, of course. By changing the subject, by avoiding the topic, by trying to convince your wife to cheer up."[2]

Silver's words may resonate with your experience. Maybe your husband changes the subject when he doesn't know what to do with it. Maybe he avoids talking cancer altogether. Or maybe you find he is continually trying to cheer you up, even when what you need most is a good cry on his shoulder.

If it had been possible, Corey would have "fixed it" by taking the burden from me. And he's not the only husband to feel this way. Steve had similar impulses when his wife was diagnosed with breast cancer at age sixty-four. But he learned it was a problem he couldn't solve. He said, "My first response is to try to fix it, but I had to remind myself many times that not everything is mine to fix."

Another husband, Dan, experienced the same feelings about his wife, Heather, when she received the diagnosis of triple negative breast cancer. He said, "I prayed and shed many tears in private asking God, 'Why? Why couldn't it have been me? She doesn't deserve this.' The song 'Rejoice in the Lord Always' would often come to mind. But how could I rejoice in this? I remember feeling angry and afraid." Dan said he worked hard to change his focus and trust that God was in control regardless of the circumstances they found themselves in.

Despite men's tendencies to want to solve problems, taking the cancer from us (and all the pain that comes with it) is not an option. I think every guy who walks through this has to do some form of soul searching as they come to grips with the fact that there is no easy way out and that this is not a problem they can fix.

Communication

Corey and I sat a long time in a Johnny's Steakhouse parking lot with the truck still running. All the extra McDonald's napkins I could find in the glove box were soaked with our snot and tears, and we wondered whether or not we could pull ourselves together enough to go in and enjoy date night.

The cause of those tears? An argument inspired by breast cancer. What in the world? Why were we having these awful arguments now when we needed each other so much? Neither of us wanted it to be this way, but we were both so stressed out and vulnerable and we didn't know how to make it better. Cancer threw us for a loop. Though we grew incredibly intimate in many ways through the mastectomy and reconstruction process, we were also blindsided by opposing thoughts and feelings that sparked friction. I don't want you to think that we argued all the time, because we definitely didn't. We had a lot of conversations during breast cancer that were really good and deepened our relationship. But some, like the one at Johnny's, ended with elevated voices, puffy eyes, and a pile of Kleenex.

You face so many difficult decisions that must be made in quick succession after a breast cancer diagnosis—all while wrestling with your mortality. Questions like these: Should I ask for a lumpectomy, even though they are recommending a mastectomy? Should I have one breast removed? Both? Should I have it (or them) reconstructed? What type of reconstruction? How large should they be? What type of implant should I go with? What about my nipples? Should I have the surgeon try to save those? Reconstruct them? Should I have them tattooed on later?

These decisions that neither of us wanted to make drove a wedge between us. I would get angry because he wasn't immediately supportive of all my choices. He would get angry because I was making all the decisions on my own and leaving him completely out of the process. And both of us did a dang poor job of articulating our frustrations in a way the other could understand.

It was miserable.

To live life utterly in love with Corey and clinging to him to get through each day and yet have a chasm between us was absolutely horrible. That chasm, made up of all the decisions that had to be made and the way we handled it, felt impossible to cross. Ugh. Cancer sucks.

If you are struggling in a similar way, rest assured you are not an anomaly. Silver puts it this way: "A breast cancer husband is surely experiencing a number of feelings—fear, sorrow, optimism, pessimism, numbness, annoyance at his wife. . . . At times you and your wife will feel frustrated with each other. The challenge, psychologists say, is to support your wife with love and companionship whether you are disclosing your feelings or keeping them inside."[3]

On the flip side of this, I think we wives can be good companions to our husbands by allowing them into the process with us, by making this cancer journey a team effort instead of doing it all on our own. I've learned that an important piece of this communication struggle is that our husbands can end up feeling pushed aside. In my case, I really didn't consider how much Corey would care about being a part of the process as I barreled through the barrage of available options. I made decisions without his input, and in doing so, I hurt him deeply. His hurt led to my frustration because I didn't understand how my actions affected him.

Apparently this is not uncommon in the world of cancer. According to a team of psychologists at Stanford Medicine, the pain, fear, and confusion endured by the cancer patient's spouse or partner is often overlooked, and the spouse can end up feeling shunted aside. But the more the spouse participates in the ongoing decision-making and treatment discussions and the more experiences the couple shares, the less likely it is that they will drift apart.[4]

Unfortunately, pushing aside your spouse (often unintentionally) is not uncommon, and it causes emotional collateral damage. Dave Willis, author of *The Naked Marriage*, says, "In marriage, there will be times when you 'step on each other's toes,' so to speak. But the really hurtful moments happen when you 'step on each other's hearts' and wound your spouse on an emotional level. There are times when one spouse might intentionally try to hurt the other, but I'm convinced that many of the most damaging wounds in marriage are inflicted unintentionally."[5]

That's what Corey and I were doing to each other—unintentionally hurting each other emotionally. Once we figured out the problem (though there was still hurt and pain to overcome), we were able to resume an intimacy in our emotional relationship that had been broken. Looking back at that part of cancer still hurts a lot. Honestly, neither of us even like to think about it, but it was an opportunity for our relationship to grow. And for that, I'm thankful.

This scenario happens all too often with couples dealing with breast cancer. Another survivor's husband, Steve, didn't feel left out of the process like my Corey, but he didn't always agree with his wife's decisions. At one point, he believed his wife was making a choice she would later regret. She decided to go flat on one side after a unilateral mastectomy, and he tried to convince her to choose reconstruction because he thought that she would eventually miss having that breast. His presumptions left her feeling hurt and unsupported. He said:

"I was concerned she would change her mind in a year or two and I knew it would be easier to pursue reconstruction now than later, so I tried to push her to rethink her decision. But what I had to remind myself about my wife is that she is an internal processor, and by the time she comes up with her answer, she has put a lot of thought and consideration into it. When she verbalizes her decision, it's done. She's not going to change her mind."

A study in the *Journal of Psychosocial Oncology* found that friction in a marriage as a result of breast cancer is not unusual. According to the study, one cause of friction is differing views about the cancer. Husbands and wives can differ in their philosophies on how to best deal with the cancer, on the extent of questions asked about treatment, and on how much they want to talk to others or explore the emotional side of the experience.[6] There are several opportunities for possible disagreements and misunderstandings during this high-stress time in our lives.

It may be hard to think about communication and the possibility of clashing opinions at the beginning of your journey when the fear and uncertainty of cancer loom over your head, but it's worthwhile to consider talking up front with your spouse about how the two of you plan to communicate and make decisions moving forward. Having a picture of how each person feels about making decisions at the beginning of the wild ride of mastectomy and breast reconstruction is better than finding yourselves at an impasse several months into it.

Grief

Losing a distinctly feminine body part is challenging in many ways. I'm a few years past cancer, and I still long for "normal" breasts sometimes. I'm sure you do too. Our men also miss our breasts. The problem that arises with a lot of guys is they are so relieved that we are past cancer and thankful we are alive that they feel guilty about longing for our natural breasts. I remember a night when it brought Corey to tears. "I just miss your boobs." I needed to be okay with him missing them. I went through a grieving process and he had to grieve as well. So if and when your hubby tells you that he misses your boobs, try to put yourself in his place and understand that this change in your body is hard for him too.

Many couples are not immune to this challenge. It rang true with Dan, who grieved his wife Heather's breasts, but he tried to keep everything in perspective. Both he and Heather miss the sensitivity of her natural breasts during intimacy, but they also believe it was worth giving up in order to give Heather the best chance at a healthy future.

An experienced anesthesiologist said, "A loving partner would be saddened not because he or she thinks breasts are the end-all and be-all of female sexuality, or that a woman's worth is related to her body parts, but rather because such surgery strikes so visibly and painfully at the heart of a lot of shared stories, intimate moments, mutual devotion, and cherished physicality."[7]

It also took Vickie's husband, Steve, a while to get used to the *new her*. He said, "It was terribly hard at first. The scar tissue was all red. It just looked like it really hurt. And even when she was healed, it still took time to get used to her new body." But in the years that have passed since Vickie's cancer experience, Steve said her *new body* has become normal.

Know that your hubby has to work through this just like you do, and that it will take time. If we can expect bumps in the road and be prepared for those steps backwards that will occur now and then, we will make our way through this journey with a healthier perspective. Grieving is a process that cannot be rushed.

Outside Support

After I received my diagnosis, a group of close friends became an invaluable support system. I could text these women any time of the day or night and trust that they would take care of any need that arose. I also had the freedom during the hard times to say, "Hey, I can't handle people today," and they would understand and give me space.

Dealing with emotions of their own, our men benefit from outside support too. Ziva Naghiyeva, an Oncology Supportive Care Services clinical social worker at Cedars-Sinai in Los Angeles, says it's important for the partners of cancer patients to have their own support. "There should be a second ring of support exclusively for these partners. They need a trusted friend, family member, or therapist as an outlet for their own feelings, which will continue to build if neglected."[8]

Corey was an elder in our church when I walked through cancer, so he had a group of guys that he already regularly met with and felt free to talk to and pray with. He also had a couple of friends who regularly checked in on him. I don't know what they talked about. I don't know how often he cried, how often he felt frustrated, or how often he was confused; I just know that he needed people to share the burden with who weren't me.

Having a support system helped previvor Rachel's husband, Eric, as well. He had a few friends he was able to confide in throughout the process. After Rachel tested positive for the BRCA2 gene mutation, he knew hard decisions were ahead. He said, "I think my struggles were with how I could support her and the ultimate decision [whether or not to undergo a prophylactic mastectomy and **oophorectomy** to diminish her high risk of breast cancer and ovarian cancer]. I knew we couldn't change genetics, so what were our options?"

Not all men have a built-in support system like Corey and Eric did, however. In *Breast Cancer Husband*, author Marc Silver notes that in many marriages, if the husband has something to talk about, his wife is the one person he feels he can talk to. "Men often don't have a clutch of good buddies who sit for hours and talk frankly about life and sex and death. If a fellow talks to anyone about these heavy topics, it's probably his spouse."[9]

This concept correlated with Brant's experience. It took some time for him to work through the variety of emotions he experienced, but it was primarily an internal process for him because so few people could truly understand what he was going through. "Post-surgery it felt very lonely as [my wife] was recovering. It was hard to not have my partner and best friend with me in the same capacity for a while."

Like the experience of breast cancer is individually unique for each woman walking through it, so it is for each husband. Different men will have different needs in regard to a place to unload and find support, but it is beneficial for everyone to have access to someone they can talk to if needed. This may be in the form of a friend, a colleague, or possibly even a breast cancer husband support group or counselor.

A Faith Perspective

Some things you just can't share with other people. Some hurts run too deep for words, and it's during hard times like cancer that many people lean into God. It's interesting that science seems to confirm that having faith through hard life events is beneficial.

When cancer enters the picture, so does anxiety. But according to Barbara Markway at *Psychology Today*, spirituality can ease anxiety in four ways: it can make you feel more hopeful, help you be more open to different ways of dealing with anxiety, improve your attitudes and behaviors to evolve naturally in a more positive direction, and change the way you view your problems.[10]

Faith can be tested in times of difficulty, but it can also grow stronger in the struggle. This was the case for Brant, who wrestled with some tough emotions. He said, "After surgery, I was definitely angry, resentful, and hurt. I withdrew a bit from my church because I knew God could lift this burden but He didn't. It took me a bit to work through this. As [my wife] Ronell healed and we reached a new normal, I worked through those feelings. I have an assurance that God is in control and that He brings peace."

Another survivor's husband, Steve, said his faith was stretched like Brant's, but he grew through cancer as well. And meditating on a key scripture passage helped him through a lot of hard times. (I love this because these verses are the very words I clung to throughout cancer.) It reads:

But now, this is what the Lord says—He who created you, Jacob, He who formed you, Israel: "Do not fear, for I have redeemed you; I have summoned you by name; you are mine. When you pass through the waters, I will be with you; and when you pass through the rivers, they will not sweep over you. When you walk through the fire, you will not be burned; the flames will not set you ablaze. For I am the Lord your God, the Holy One of Israel, your Savior." (Isaiah 43:1–3 [NIV])

Faith in a power higher than himself helped survivor Rachel's husband, Eric, as well. He doesn't know how he and Rachel could have gotten through the results of her BRCA2 gene mutation and all that came with it without their faith. He said, "We will never understand during this life why God lets us go through some things. Maybe it's to walk with a friend going through the same thing, or to encourage a husband, or to give advice. But I know God's plan is perfect. Period. His faithfulness is evident today, and I don't thank God enough for each day we have together."

Faith is not a piece of every person's story, and people make it to the other side of hard things without it. But I have found that those with a measure of faith receive added support for the journey.

As Married Couples, We're in This Together

I'm not a man, obviously, so everything I've written in this chapter about a man's perspective comes through a female's worldview. If you want to dive more deeply into a man's perspective on breast cancer, I highly recommend picking up a copy of Marc Silver's book *Breast Cancer Husband*. But in the meantime, I hope my words have given you some understanding of the road your spouse or loved one travels with you and perhaps provided you both with sound advice of where to avoid or work through possible snags in your relationship during this difficult time.

Advice for Husbands by Husbands

- "Go to as many of your wife's appointments with her as you can. It's somewhat uncomfortable watching the doctor touch your wife in front of you, but it's uncomfortable for her as well, and being there for support is a good thing." —Dan

- "Love her more than you ever have. Think about the changes she is enduring and how they may affect her image of herself. Then love her more. Tell her she is beautiful, hot, sexy. Whatever it takes." —Eric

- "Be careful not to give her the idea that you aren't supporting her, but don't be afraid to talk through the decisions that need to be made." —Steve

- "Do the little things. Sometimes all it takes is holding her hand while she sleeps." —Eric

- "Pray. Pray together and pray separate. Praying together is something I don't do well, but I think it's important." —Steve

- "Stay positive. Listen. Be patient. Be solid. And stock the liquor cabinet." —Brant

Resources

1. Powell, Robert. "Inside the Male Brain: Why Do Men Behave the Way They Do?" *Today*, November 4, 2016. https://www.today.com/health/inside-male-brain-why-do-men-behave-way-they-do-t104668.

2. Silver, Marc. *Breast Cancer Husband: How to Help Your Wife (And Yourself) Through Diagnosis, Treatment and Beyond*. Emmaus, PA: Rodale Books, 2004.

3. Ibid.

4. Kneier, Andrew; Kelly, Patricia T.; and Rosenbaum, Ernest H. "When Your Spouse Has Cancer." Stanford Medicine, accessed December 2, 2019. http://med.stanford.edu/survivingcancer/cancer-and-stress/when-your-spouse-has-cancer.html.

5. Willis, Dave. "4 Things You Should Never Ever Do in Marriage." MarriageToday.com, May 15, 2018. https://marriagetoday.com/marriagehelp/4-things-never-ever-marriage/.

6. Zahlis, Ellen H., and Lewis, Frances M. 2010. "Coming to Grips with Breast Cancer: The Spouse's Experience with His Wife's First Six Months." *Journal of Psychosocial Oncology* 28, no. 1: 79–97. https://www.ncbi.nlm.nih.gov/pmc/articles/PMC2856107/.

7. T, Anesthesioboist. "The Grief Men Face When Their Wives Undergo Mastectomies." KevinMD.com, July 8, 2010. https://www.kevinmd.com/blog/2010/07/grief-men-face-wives-undergo-mastectomies.html.

8. Cedars-Sinai Staff. "What to Do When the Woman in Your Life Has Breast Cancer." Cedars-Sinai Blog, October 29, 2017. https://www.cedars-sinai.org/blog/woman-life-breast-cancer.html.

9. Marc Silver, *Breast Cancer Husband*.

10. Markway, Barbara. "4 Powerful Ways Spirituality Can Ease Anxiety and Depression." *Psychology Today*, March 31, 2016. https://www.psychologytoday.com/us/blog/living-the-questions/201603/4-powerful-ways-spirituality-can-ease-anxiety-and-depression.

Chapter 10

Don't Forget to Include Your Kids: They May Not Ask Questions, but They Have Them

"I was scared when my mom had cancer. I was hoping she was not going to die."
—Lewis Harms, 9 years old

"Did you have your appointment today?"

It was the evening of biopsy day and I was driving Carter home from basketball practice. My oldest is a man of few words, just like his daddy. He doesn't ask a lot of questions, and he rarely offers his heart. So when words come out of his mouth, I listen. I knew those six words were a big deal.

Underneath that question was the deeper question I know he couldn't bring himself to ask: "Do you have cancer?" More than anything, I wanted to ease his worry. I wanted to say, "Everything's a-okay. I just had a simple little procedure, and I'm all clear." But

I didn't know. And I didn't want to give him false hope. "I had the biopsy. It went smoothly, and I'm feeling okay, but we don't have the results yet," was the best that I could do.

The next day it was affirmed that cancer had indeed invaded my left breast. I could answer Carter's question now, but how? How does a mom do that? What's the best way to break your child's heart? Over ice cream after supper? During a commercial break in the NBA game? In the dark quiet of his room at bedtime? Ugh. There is no good time to tell your kids you have cancer.

Corey and I decided it would be best to call a family meeting (the meeting I described in the introduction of this book). Looking back, I still think that was the best way to bring our kids into our new cancer world, but it wasn't easy.

Your family is no doubt different from mine, and you have to do things in the way that works for you. Maybe that's telling your kids one-on-one, maybe it's over dinner, or maybe it's at a family meeting like us. I can't answer that for you. But I do believe there are some thoughts all parents should consider while traveling this crappy road.

To Shelter or to Share

My mama instinct is to protect my kids. I'm sure yours is too. But sometimes protecting them is not an option. And sometimes sheltering our children from the hurt isn't the right answer, even if it is an option. When hard things smack us from behind and knock the wind out of us, the best answer is not always to figure out how to shield our kids from pain but instead to decipher how to help them walk through the pain with us. Our January 21st family meeting was awful. It was heart-breaking. It was a conversation no parent ever wants to have with their children. But it was necessary. And it was the beginning of growth in my boys that would not have happened without cancer. We never would have chosen it, of course, but I see all three of my boys on the other side of cancer, stronger and more compassionate than ever before.

I can't give you a step-by-step guide for walking your kids through cancer and breast reconstruction with you, just like I couldn't for walking you through the grief of losing your breasts. But I think the key word here is *with*. The depth of the *with* differs depending on varying ages and maturity of kids. For instance, your two-year-old and four-year-old are probably more suited to benefit from that motherly sheltering instinct. But those older kids? I am convinced they need in on this. Again, the amount they need to know varies with things like age, maturity, gender, and personality, but open communication is vital.

According to the American Psychological Association, taking a proactive stance and discussing difficult events in age-appropriate language can help children feel safer and more secure.[1] In my experience as an adult, when I am armed with information, I feel more secure. So it makes sense that my kids will operate similarly.

From the day I found out I had cancer until the day (a week later) I met with a surgeon, I struggled with an almost disabling amount of fear. I prayed constantly, asking God to take the fear away, and it was the most intense concern I have ever battled with in my mind and spirit. But after sitting with my surgeon and creating a game plan, the fear began to ease. And here's the deal—nothing had changed. I still had the same cancer I had before that appointment. But now I possessed information for the battle.

If knowing the ins and outs of Mom's cancer treatment will ease our kids' fears, then figure out a way to keep the conversation going—this is where being proactive comes in. We must study our children to know what they can handle and share with them according to their needs and abilities to process the information.

According to Caroline Knorr of Common Sense Media, every child brings his or her own sensitivities, temperament, experience, and other individual traits to any conversation, and it's essential to take those into consideration.[2] It's important to understand a bit of how kids perceive the world in each phase of development to provide guidance in presenting information in an age-appropriate way. Maybe for you, this means regular, scheduled family meetings to talk about what's going on. Maybe it means acting as a comforter to your fearful children. And maybe it's something in between.

Breast cancer is awkward and hard to grasp for boys making their way through puberty. What teenage boy wants to have to think about, much less talk about, his mom's boobs? But that's where my cancer was. I didn't get to choose where the cancer showed up in my body. My kids had no choice but to get over that awkwardness hurdle. And in the long run, I think it was good for them. Chances are that one day they will have a wife or friend or mother-in-law who will go through this same thing, and they will have some preparation for it.

Corey and I decided to be as open as possible about the things that were happening to my body. We kept them informed, but we also gave them the option to say "Too much information. Please stop talking now" when it was too much to take.

For the most part, our teenagers were interested in what happened at my appointments, but they did draw the line at nipple tattoos. The night before my tattoo appointment, we offered to show the older two boys photos of nipple tattoos so they would know what this step of the process was like. They turned that offer down flat. I guess some things they just don't want to know.

We were more careful with the information we shared with our second grader. We primarily made ourselves available to him whenever he needed and answered his questions in language he could understand. It worked well for us.

But like I've mentioned before, you should handle this process according to your own family's needs, and *you* know your children best. Survivor Ronell, who was diagnosed at age forty-two, was very intentional about keeping her older kids in the loop. She and her husband, Brant, decided to give a dinner table update every time she had an appointment or received new information. But they chose to explain the actual mastectomy and reconstruction procedures to their kids one-on-one, because they knew each child held a different capacity to handle the information. Ronell described the surgery to her son, Brady, by using an analogy of an orange split in half with the insides scooped out and replaced with Jell-O.

"He looked at me like, 'What the heck? Are you kidding me?' But I felt like he needed to know to appreciate that this was a major surgery."

Her fifteen-year-old daughter, McKenna, was able to have a deeper conversation. And because of the openness throughout the process, Ronell and her daughter are even able to crack "cleavage" jokes on occasion (now that they are past the scary stuff). Ronell said, "I think adults discount what kids can handle and what can be helpful for them to know. And I strongly believe information can weed out fear. I feel like my kids needed information so they would not be fearful."

Many women have grown children at diagnosis. Most of the women mentioned in this book are younger (under fifty years of age). But as we age, our breast cancer risk increases, so a lot of women are tasked with breaking the cancer news to grown children.

This was the case with survivor Jane, whose son was twenty-eight when she was diagnosed. Because he didn't live nearby, she made a hard phone call to give him the news, fearful of how it would affect him. "As moms, we never get over wanting to protect our children," she said. The next day, he drove eighty miles and showed up at her door with a new board game to help take her mind off of her upcoming medical consultation. He spent the night at her house and hugged his mama tight before leaving her the next day. Instead of needing comfort and assurance like a small child, he needed to make sure his mom received comfort and reassurance from him. A biomedical engineer, her son stayed involved and asked questions throughout her cancer, doing a lot of his own research to know what was going on in his mom's body and how the treatments would work to heal her.

Younger kids obviously can't handle the depth of information teens and adult children can, but previvor Krystal made sure her kids knew the basics of her procedures. "They knew Mommy had a high risk of getting cancer and that because of that, she was going to lose her boobs, and the doctors were going to build her new ones." They were less concerned with details than with just knowing their mom was going to be okay.

When and Where to Talk

Keeping our kids informed is important, but it's also imperative to consider when and where to do so. Children who are old enough to understand what's going on likely want to be a part of the journey, but they may not come right out and say it. When my quiet teenager asked, "Did you have your appointment today?" he was inviting himself in to this challenge in my life. Look for cues in the words of your own children to help you know just how to bring them along on this journey.

I took advantage of the times my boys were open to conversation. It wasn't about when it was convenient for me but *when it was necessary for them*. My youngest is never afraid to tell me what's on his mind, but my teens are different. Both Carter and Owen mastered the art of one-syllable answers at a young age, so over the years I've learned how to watch for their I'm-ready-to-talk cues. I knew that pushing them to talk when they weren't up for it would ultimately push them away. But I also knew they needed an outlet to process their thoughts and questions verbally, and it was up to me to recognize when they were ready to do that.

Our conversations usually happened in the car (like that ride home from basketball practice) and at bedtime. Long before cancer, we had a bedtime back-scratching routine. Every night I spent a few minutes at their bedside, scratching their backs. Aside from the weeks when I was healing from surgery, I continued this nightly bedtime ritual throughout cancer, and that is often when the questions would come. Some nights they were silent, but other nights in the dark calm of the moonlight, their hearts opened up and poured out through their words. These were rarely long, deep conversations, but they were enough to give my boys peace of mind for the moment. And peace of mind for the moment is what this mama wanted more than anything for her boys as they drifted off to sleep.

Survivor Ronell also worked to keep the communication lines open with her kids. "My son, Brady (twelve), was sort of standoffish about it at first, but he was more apt to talk one-on-one. Every parent knows the magic of the car ride, and he had weekly allergy shots that required a forty-minute drive together. Alone in the car, that's when he would talk to me."

Fifteen-year-old McKenna approached it a little differently. She kept her thoughts and emotions locked up pretty tight after diagnosis, while Ronell gently (but persistently) worked to keep the conversation going. In the end, a connection the mom and daughter shared over MRI experiences allowed McKenna to open up. Having had an injury that required the teen to have an MRI prior to her mom's diagnosis, McKenna realized she had some valuable insight to offer her mom and that she didn't have to be a silent spectator to this hard thing her mom was going through. From then on she became willing and interested in talking things out.

Survivor Heather's experience wasn't a matter of sharing details but about providing her children with needed comfort. Her youngest child was a preschooler at the time of her diagnosis. Her daughter was primarily concerned about whether or not Mom was going to be okay; she didn't need details, she just needed reassurance that they were going to make it through this. Heather said she knew all her kids were fearful, though they didn't express it in those words. "They continually just wanted to be reassured that I was okay."

In contrast, previvor Rachel's kids were so young when she tested positive for the BRCA 2 gene mutation that she and her husband, Eric, chose not to tell them at all. In fact, her sister took her kids in for a period of time after surgery, so for the most part, the children weren't even exposed to their mom's discomfort.

Your family may function in a similar way to a family I've mentioned in this chapter, or it may be totally different. The important thing isn't to get this perfectly right but to be aware of our kids' needs to receive information and talk *with* them as they wrestle with questions and fears. (See sidebar for suggestions for keeping your children in the loop.)

Parenting-through-Cancer Suggestions

- Keep your kids' schoolteachers, counselors, and coaches in the loop.
- Keep their friends' parents in the loop too.
- Be a student of your children. Study them to become aware of how much information they need and what level of depth is appropriate to share with them.
- Don't underestimate your kids' ability to handle hard things. Keeping them completely out of the loop is probably not the right answer.
- Live openly enough that they are comfortable asking questions.
- Be available and willing to answer their questions.
- Don't be afraid to let them see you be weak. Our vulnerability opens up the door for our kids to be vulnerable with us.
- Don't hide your tears. Crying in front of your kids might just allow them to feel vulnerable enough to cry with you and share their thoughts and feelings.

- Reassure them. It's okay for our kids to know that we struggle with fear and uncertainty, but it's also important for us to reassure them that we are in this together.
- Think about what you are going to say before you have a hard conversation. Practice in front of a mirror if that helps.
- Have a loved one take your kids shopping to buy you a pre-surgery gift. It makes them feel like they are doing something for you. Lewis picked out a stuffed animal for me to take to the hospital.

Retaining Some Normalcy

After diagnosis, I knew our lives were forever changed and that the coming months would be exceedingly hard on all five of us. With that in mind, I started considering specific things I could do to help retain some normalcy in the boys' lives. One of my first moves was to send an email to all of their friends' parents begging them not to get weird (cancer tends to make people weird) and asking them to keep letting their kids come hang out in our home. You see, up to that point, we'd always had an open-door policy at our house. Friends were in and out all the time. Sometimes they stayed for a little while, sometimes they joined us for dinner, and sometimes I found one on a couch or the floor the next morning. I didn't want that to change. Thankfully it didn't, and I'm forever grateful to the parents who obliged my request.

This principle of retaining normalcy held true for survivor Ronell's family's life as well. By recruiting her dad as the "family Uber driver," her kids continued to make it to all of their practices, classes, and games. And by taking people up on their offers to provide meals, Ronell was freed up to attend a lot of the kids' events when she felt well enough, making life feel more normal.

Being "normal" is tough. Some things have to change when Mom is thrown into the crazy world of mastectomy and breast reconstruction, but it is worth it to think about the things in life that are possible to keep the same (or nearly the same) as before cancer and work hard to keep them that way.

When You Are Genetically Predisposed to Breast Cancer (BRCA1, BRCA2 Gene Mutations)

My cancer was not genetic. I'll never know what caused it. Several people thought they knew and were so kind (read the sarcasm here) as to send me articles telling me the things I should have been doing to prevent cancer: I got cancer because I ate red meat. I got cancer because I didn't eat enough broccoli and blueberries. I got cancer because I ate processed foods. I got cancer because I drank cow's milk . . . If I chose to believe all those things, I would've drowned in guilt for not preventing this disease from entering my body. But I digress.

I will never know what thing or combination of things caused my cancer, but because of modern medical technology, some women can trace their cancer back to a tiny little gene mutation. This is a good thing, but it's not an easy thing. It's good because some women discover their mutation before cancer invades and are able to undergo preventative surgery prior to a cancer diagnosis. But it's hard too. Not only because the surgeries required are extremely taxing, but because if a woman is found to have the gene mutation, her children have a good chance of having it too. This poses an extra challenge. When and how should they break the news to their daughters that they may someday have to go through this too? And what about their sons, who have the potential to pass the gene to their children?

These are questions those with this gene mutation must face and eventually share with their children. Previvor Krystal said she was grateful she found out about the mutation after marriage and having kids because it was easier to make the decision to go through with a bilateral mastectomy and talk about a potential hysterectomy when she knew her family was complete. But knowing that her elementary-age kids could also have the gene mutation, she often considers at what age she will have the hard conversation with them.

Previvor Rachel wrestles with the same issue for her three daughters and one son. Because this gene mutation isn't linked to childhood cancers and insurance doesn't allow testing until age eighteen, she's not in a hurry to tell them, but she doesn't yet know when the right time will be. She said:

> A couple of our kids have some struggles with anxiety, so I don't want to tell them early and give them something to worry about. I want to wait until they are old enough to really understand what it means and the options they will face. I will probably encourage them to not get tested right away—it can have insurance (especially life) eligibility consequences. I was glad I didn't get my results until I was at a stage of life that I was ready to do something about it. I probably would have just worried about it and been super paranoid had I known earlier.

Though the risk for breast cancer in male carriers of the gene mutation is considerably lower than a female's risk (1 to 10 percent in men compared to 50 to 85 percent in women[3]), it is generally recommended that boys get tested. They are just as likely as their sisters to carry the genetic mutation, according to the Cancer Treatment Centers of America. Genetic counselor Melanie Corbman believes it's beneficial for males to get tested because they are potential carriers who can pass the gene to their children and because having the gene mutation increases their own risk of developing other types of cancer, including prostate cancer, pancreatic cancer, and melanoma.[4]

No formula exists to tell you how or when to inform your children that they may carry the gene mutation. It's not about a right or a wrong time but about your preferences and knowledge of your child's personality and whether or not he or she is mature enough to handle the information.

Looking Back

It's been a few years now since all the cancer stuff happened at our house. I know that a stage I invasive ductal carcinoma diagnosis has a 99 percent five-year survival rate, and that brings me comfort. But I also know enough people for whom cancer returned (including dear Jodi, who first appears in Chapter 2 of this book and has since passed on) that I live my life with a clear understanding that I am not promised a tomorrow. And my boys have a more sober view of life and death than most teenagers do.

Because our family was forced to look at life in a new way through cancer, and because we did it together, we now live life more fully together. Once you face death, you are more motivated to live life. We're normal people and our week-to-week life probably looks similar to a lot of middle-class Americans, but we *do* things together. Big things. Things I probably wouldn't have taken the time for without cancer. We spent a week at a hotel in Daytona Beach the year after cancer because I decided a cancer diagnosis deserves a trip to the ocean. We didn't even have a plan while we were there. We just swam, played round after round of mini golf, and ate pancakes at a Denny's on Thanksgiving Day. We've gone backpacking twice since cancer. A few summers ago we took our oldest two to Haiti on a mission trip. And in the fall of 2018, we got a puppy—which I was never, *ever* going to do. (The jury is still out on whether or not that last move was a good one.)

Thankfully, I didn't have the hard physical task of trying to parent through the sick and tired feelings of chemotherapy. And I didn't have to lose my hair or keep "momming" through the exhaustion of radiation. Women who've walked that road are rock stars. But any breast cancer diagnosis or positive genetic mutation test, regardless of the specifics of treatment, changes your life and the lives of your children. Suddenly tomorrow is not a given. The thought of loss grips your mind and wreaks havoc with your emotions. It's a really, really hard thing, but it's not all bad.

I'm thankful for my new perspective and for the ways my boys were forced to mature through that hard year. I'm now proactively parenting post-cancer. And I love my life. My hope for you is that you will also learn to find joy and live fully *with* your family.

Resources

1. "How to Talk to Children about Difficult News." American Psychological Association, April 13, 2020. Accessed May 11, 2020. https://www.apa. org/helpcenter/talking-to-children.
2. Knorr, Caroline. "Explaining the News to Our Kids." Common Sense Media, March 12, 2020. https://www.commonsensemedia.org/blog/ explaining-the-news-to-our-kids.
3. "If Cancer Runs in Your Family . . . Information about BRCA Testing for Men," Facing Our Risk of Cancer Empowered (FORCE), accessed May 14, 2020. https://www.facingourrisk.org/understand-ing-brca-and-hboc/publications/documents/Info%20for%20Men%20 Flyer%207.16.14.pdf.
4. "What Does BRCA Gene Mutation Mean for Men?" Cancer Treatment Centers of America, June 1, 2017. https://www.cancercenter.com/ community/blog/2017/06/what-does-a-brca-gene-mutation-mean-for -men.

Chapter 11

Humor in the Hurting: Sometimes Laughter Is the Best Medicine

"Humor is an antidote to all ills."
—Patch Adams

F%&# Cancer. Kill Karen.

I might have spit out my coffee when I scrolled through my new friend's Facebook page. Alex gave her cancer that infamous girl name, Karen, and took care of business with the f-word and hilarious "Kill Karen" memes. It made me laugh out loud.

I am not a cussing person. In fact, before becoming a first-time dog owner last year, I didn't even swear inside my head. But I challenge you to keep your thoughts G-rated while training a puppy to stop eating his own poop. I'm pretty sure it's not possible. Though it's a rare day that you will hear any swearing in our house, I am a firm believer that when you get the cancer call, a slip of the f-bomb is 100 percent acceptable. Corey agrees. In fact, he keeps a running list of circumstances in which he believes that word is wholly appropriate.

Just for fun, here's his list of Top Five Acceptable Usages of the F-Bomb, in no particular order:

1. Getting left on Mars by yourself. (If you haven't seen the movie *The Martian*, put it on your list.)

2. Being placed on the front lines of a war. (I have a strong aversion to listening to the f-word in most movies, but it felt right in *Hacksaw Ridge* and *Saving Private Ryan*.)

3. Zombie apocalypse. (Um, if a zombie is coming after me to eat my brain, "Oh, crap" is not going to cut it.)

4. Realizing midair that your parachute won't open. (A good chance the f-bomb will be your final word in this situation.)

5. Cancer diagnosis.

I love Jesus, and I want my actions and my words to point people toward God, but when Alex posted a photo of herself with a "Kill Karen" bracelet and an "F Cancer" shirt, it brought me joy and laughter. (She loves Jesus too, by the way. She just also understands that some situations call for strong words.)

I'm sure some of you think this cuss word business isn't funny and that I should get on my knees and confess my effing sin, and others are like, "What's the big deal? That's one of my favorite descriptors." My point is not to argue the validity or vulgarity of swearing but to simply state that when you have cancer, saying bad words and laughing at things that aren't funny can be a helpful way to get through it with at least some of your sanity intact.

But enough about why I deem the f-bomb useful and funny. Let's talk about the overall value of humor and laughter in the midst of serious illness.

Physiological Benefits

Did you know that our bodies actually produce painkilling hormones called endorphins in response to laughter? A belly laugh literally increases the production of T cells, and T cells are an important part of the healing process. Dr. William C. Sheil Jr. describes them as "soldiers who search out and destroy the targeted invaders."[1] How cool is that? The simple act of laughing actually produces physical results in our bodies.

Hunter (Patch) Adams, MD, the man whose life inspired the 1998 movie *Patch Adams*, understood this truth decades ago. In 1971, he started a free hospital where thousands of patients received humor-infused care over the course of the twelve years it was open. It later evolved into the Gesundheit! Institute, which is a nonprofit organization that offers services like "humanitarian clowning" trips to hospitals and educational programs designed to teach medical students how to relate compassionately to their patients. Though Adams is considered by some in the medical community as radical in the way he approaches medical treatment, he has science to back up the validity of humor-infused treatment. He continues to devote his life to expanding the Gesundheit! Institute and sharing his passion with others.[2]

During my breast cancer year, a group of friends and I kept an ongoing group text thread. We had nights when we all sat in our separate homes laughing until tears ran down our faces as we shot inappropriate "funny-not-funny" jokes to each other through cyber-space. In fact, at the end of one such night, my friend Deanna's husband sent me a video of her laughing uncontrollably as she took part in the texting hilarity. Deanna previously walked through the cancer of her nine-year-old daughter, having fought hard together to beat a 20 percent chance of survival. If she (who knows the depth of the pain of cancer) can find laughter in the face of it, anyone can. (By the way, her daughter overcame the odds and is now a wonderfully sweet college student.)

The instance I remember most clearly happened on a night I will call "The Oreo Symposium." I'd just discovered Mega Stuf Oreos and we were discussing the appropriate amount of filling for the delicious little sandwich cookie. Somehow during the course of this conversation, my breasts became Oreos and the discussion morphed into the appropriate amount of filling for *my* Oreos. In this bizarre world of breast reconstruction, deciding how much filling to put in your boob(s) is a real decision that has to be made. Inserting some humor into the thought process (like the filling of an Oreo) makes it a little less heartbreaking.

As an experienced Oreo eater, I believe the Double-Stuf is cookie perfection. Single-Stuf leaves me a little dissatisfied, and Mega Stuf is just too sweet. But if I had to describe the final product of Kim's Boob Oreos, I would definitely say I landed on the Single-Stuf side. I didn't think more *filling* would look quite right on my 5-foot-3-inch 110-pound frame, and I really didn't want to get to the other side of cancer and feel self-conscious about people checking out my big, new Oreos.

Thinking back, that whole process was unbelievably sad. I mean, we all just want to keep our God-given cancer-free boobs, but we can't all do that. We should totally cry about that. We should lean into that sadness and allow ourselves to mourn the loss. But we should also laugh. Laughter and tears can both have a part in our cancer story if we let them. And knowing that laughter has physiological benefits in healing, I work at finding the humor whenever I can.

Psychological Benefits

Humor and laughter not only have physical benefits but provide emotional and intellectual benefits as well. Cancer is a highly stressful experience—there is no way around it. When we are under stress, our bodies produce high levels of cortisol, which the Mayo Clinic describes as the primary stress hormone.[3] Cortisol often increases dramatically in high-stress situations.

For instance, when you get a phone call from your child that he was in a car accident, your cortisol is likely to shoot through the roof.

But when you make it to the end of the day and that child is safe at home, asleep in his bed, those cortisol levels naturally decrease. Under the long-term stress of events like cancer, cortisol levels tend to stay elevated for extended periods of time, which can lead to a number of ancillary problems like anxiety, depression, digestive problems, headaches, heart disease, sleep issues, weight gain, and memory impairment—not a fun list.

Laughter can't solve all of these problems or magically make a person emotionally stable, but it has proven to lower cortisol levels and bring the body to a more relaxed state. In *Time* magazine, Dr. Lee Berk explains that laughter shuts down the release of cortisol and triggers the production of feel-good neurochemicals like dopamine. He describes laughter as the yin to stress's yang.[4]

After sharing my diagnosis with our boys, we wanted to be sure they were in a good psychological state before we sent them back to school. We broke the news to them on a Thursday evening and let them play hooky from school on Friday. We didn't know how long it would take for the news to sink in and didn't want them to be stuck in a classroom with the urge to cry or scream or punch a wall. So we had a lazy morning at home and went out for bowling and ice cream in the afternoon. I didn't know anything about the relation of laughter to endorphins and T cells and cortisol at that time, but my mama instincts told me that we needed to have a lighthearted family day. We needed to do something that would reinforce that Mom was still Mom, even if cancer had entered the picture. So while their friends sat in algebra and English class, we took turns repeatedly tossing a heavy ball down a long lane and waiting for it to come back through a giant shark head ball return machine.

To be honest, that day didn't feel very lighthearted. I spent a lot of time swallowing down large quantities of fear. But the hours passed much faster doing something fun together than if we had tried to push through our normal routine. The day was void of belly laughs, but we did have some giggles and a measure of joy. And we got to the end of that day feeling a little less stressed out than when we started.

Incorporating Laughter into the Pain

It's easier to talk about the benefits of humor in healing than to actually incorporate humor into a heartbreaking situation. Where do we start? What should humor in the hurting look like? My close friends and hubby kept tabs on me and made sure I balanced the happy with the sad. My friend Alex started a Facebook page to connect with others and share hilarious memes. Your strategy may take a different form. If you struggle to think of how to bring some laughter into the pain, I suggest making a list of activities and things that make you happy.

The following are ten ideas to kickstart your "laughter therapy list":

1. Watch old sitcoms that made you laugh when you were a kid. (I know Bill Cosby turned out to be a gross dude, but I can still watch old episodes of *The Cosby Show* and laugh while I reminisce about my childhood.)

2. Compile a list of your favorite funny movies and have them readily available for a day when you need a little pick-me-up.

3. Go to the park and play like you did when you were a kid. (When's the last time you slid down a twisty slide?)

4. Print funny pictures and display them around your home or office.

5. Take your dog to an open field and play Frisbee (or borrow a friend's dog if you don't have one). Dogs can be great stress relievers (*after* they learn not to eat their poop).

6. Buy a joke book. Here's a joke to get you started: "What did the fish say when he hit a wall? Dam!" (My kids don't think it's very funny, but I find it hilarious.)

7. Go to the zoo and watch the monkeys.

8. Have a pillow fight with your kids.

9. Take up laughter yoga. (This is a real thing, and you might even be able to find classes in your neighborhood.)

10. Build a fire and make some gooey s'mores.

These were just a few ideas, but you can take it from here. Try to be creative, but also don't forget that even a simple activity can give you something to look forward to and help you to de-stress.

The Joy and Pain Connection

One thing I've learned over the course of my adult life is that deep joy rarely comes without deep pain. And when I look back at hard things I've walked through and wonder "How in the world was I able to laugh in the midst of that?" I remind myself that because of the depth of the pain, the depth of the joy is greater. I can laugh hard through such heartbreaking events precisely because I can cry hard through such heartbreaking events. It's like a teeter-totter at the park—you can't reach the highest height without also reaching the lowest low. The two opposites are pieces of the same whole. I think this is how joy and pain work as well—as two pieces of a whole. Think back to the last time that you laughed until you cried. I bet there's a good chance that underneath that laughter, there was a dollop of pain.

When I take inventory of my life now compared to my life before cancer, I can honestly say I have more joy in the after. I lived a happy pre-cancer life. I had a super awesome husband, fantastic kids, and the best extended family you can imagine. I had a supportive church family, many friends, and the dream job (minus the dream salary) of staying home and freelancing in my spare time. It was a good life.

But after walking through the pain of cancer, forced to look death in the face, that happy life became a deeply satisfying happy life. I laugh often. I enjoy nights of watching a *Parks and Rec* episode for the millionth time. I appreciate the giant boy shoes that clutter up my entryway. These things bring me such great joy because I know it's a gift that I am here to experience them. I live with a healthy understanding of the fact that I don't have an infinite number of breaths left to take. I'm now healthy and strong, and five-plus years cancer free.

But I know that not everyone makes it. And I know that though it's not likely, cancer could invade my body again. With this perspective in my life, appreciation of the little things is so much more, and the joy I experience is deeper. And the laughter? The laughter comes easy.

Humor versus heartache. Grief versus joy. I think we will live fuller, more contented lives if we understand that all of these things work together to make us whole. One of my favorite book quotes of all time is from a novel called *A Tree Grows in Brooklyn*. Betty Smith writes, "There had to be the dark and muddy waters so that the sun could have something to background its flashing glory."[5]

If I have to encounter dark and muddy waters to experience the flashing glory, by all means, bring on the water. And while those waters are muddy, I will make sure to put on my galoshes and take the time to jump in the puddles in search of a bit of laughter.

A Word of Caution

Humor and laughter bring lightness to the journey, but I have a word of caution for those of you who are reading this as supporters of someone going through this process. Though humor is important and holds actual healing properties, it is key to take the humor cues from the one who has cancer. Encourage her to laugh, encourage her to do lighthearted, ease-your-worry kind of things like swinging at the park or watching *Paul Blart: Mall Cop*, but don't force it. I know from experience that some days just aren't funny. Some days are for tears, not laughter.

My friends and I had a relationship where I could tell them when I wasn't in a funny mood and they would comply. Sometimes a round of texts would start and I would have to say, "I love you ladies, but not today. I can't do it today." If your cancer friend says something similar with her words or actions, follow her lead and be what she needs you to be that day. It might be a *sit and cry over coffee* day instead of a *laugh at the absurdity of rebuilt breasts* day.

If you are reading this as an acquaintance of someone going through breast reconstruction and mastectomy, or maybe even a "second-tier" friend, don't be the one to initiate the humor. If you aren't in the inner circle, saying funny things will likely come off as hurtful, not as humorous. I know this from experience. When people I didn't know very well came up to me and lightheartedly said things like, "At least you get a boob job," or "Lucky you, you get to choose the size of your boobs," it made me a little angry. (And yes, people really did say things like that.) Joking about this experience is an earned right. If you haven't shared your life with someone, you don't get to joke about cancer with them.

A Final Thought about Humor in the Hurting

Some days you will feel like you will never laugh again, like those hard days when the physical pain is overwhelming or the emotional roller-coaster is making you sick to your stomach. That's okay. Be sad. Cry it out. Sleep all day. Watch a depressing movie that fits your mood. Just don't get stuck in that place. Give yourself grace on the bad days, but love yourself enough to strive to see the joy and laughter that can come even in the hardest of life's circumstances.

Resources

1. Sheil, William C., Jr. "Medical Definition of T Cell." MedicineNet.com, updated December 27, 2018. https://www.medicinenet.com/script/main/art.asp?articlekey=11300.

2. Stout, David. "Scientist at Work: Patch Adams; Doctor in a Clown Suit Battles Ills of His Profession." *New York Times*, December 15, 1998. https://www.nytimes.com/1998/12/15/health/scientist-work-patch-adams-doctor-clown-suit-battles-ills-his-profession.html.

3. Mayo Clinic Staff. "Chronic Stress Puts Your Health at Risk." Mayo Clinic, March 19, 2019. https://www.mayoclinic.org/healthy-lifestyle/stress-management/in-depth/stress/art-20046037.

4. Heid, Markham. "You Asked: Does Laughing Have Real Health Benefits?" *Time*, November 19, 2014. https://time.com/3592134/laughing-health-benefits/.

5. Smith, Betty. *A Tree Grows in Brooklyn*. New York: Harper and Brothers, 1943.

Afterword

My boobs were recalled in 2019. How's that for the ending of this story?

Here's the thing. The cancer story doesn't ever really *end*. Once you've had it, it takes up permanent residence in the back of your mind. In my experience, I have many days when it's happy to stay there, hidden in a box in a dusty old corner of my brain. But some days. Oh, some days it sneaks out of that box and tries to cut off my oxygen.

Like the day Owen told me he had a weird lump on his neck. My first thought? *My boy has cancer. Oh Lord, don't let my boy have cancer. Bring my cancer back, but don't give it to my baby.* Well, that lump disappeared a few days later. Probably a swollen lymph node connected to a cold. But the point is, prior to cancer, my brain never would have made the leap from "Mom, can you look at this lump on my neck?" to *Oh my word, my sixteen-year-old has cancer.*

Then there's the day I learned my boobs were recalled. So many cancer emotions resurfaced. But how funny is that scenario? (Funny in a morbid sort of way.) I had my breasts removed because of cancer, and the implants that took their place were linked to causing cancer. The day I learned this, I got really mad and blasted Alanis Morrissette in my minivan. You know the song: "It's like rain on your wedding day. It's a free ride when you already paid . . ." My circumstances were far more ironic than any of the things she sings about in "Ironic," but it still felt good to belt out the lyrics with her. I let myself sit in that anger for a couple days, and then I released it and resigned myself to the fact that a surgeon was going to cut into my boobies again.

So I went under the knife in December 2019—almost four years after my cancer diagnosis. I had those cancer-causing boobs swapped out for non-cancer-causing ones in a pretty minor surgery compared to my original mastectomy and reconstruction.

In the weeks leading up to my "swap-out surgery," I wondered if all the pain and heartache would come flooding back when I put on that silly gown and those blue booties, or when I smelled that distinct hospital smell and waited in a tiny little pre-op room with Corey. I dreaded the burst of emotions I knew might push their way to the surface in the form of tears and shortness of breath as they wheeled me back to the operating room. But you know what? I was totally calm the whole time. I wasn't fearful or stricken by memories that made me cry. And I thank God for that because He always seems to provide peace beyond my understanding when I need it most. He walked me through boob-swap day just as He walked me through all the hard days that came before it.

As I write this, I'm three weeks out from that surgery. I have two new scars on the underside of my breasts, but I'm feeling pretty good. And do you want to know a secret? I like these boobs better. Who gets to say that? Who gets to say, "Well, my first set of fake boobs were okay, but I really like the shape of my second set better." Of course, I would prefer my original boobs. The ones God gave me. The ones that had feeling and nipples and were void of scars. But that option is not on the table. So I choose to focus on the silver lining. And the silver lining is that I really like the shape of these boobs.

I hope that your boobs don't get recalled. I hope your first cancer diagnosis is the only one you ever have to face. I hope your radiation scars heal and the cancer fatigue works its way out of your system. But most of all, regardless of the variety of unpleasant aftereffects that you will surely face, I hope you come out on the other side with a beautiful perspective of the precious value of life. A perspective that is impossible to achieve without walking through hard things.

I would love to sit across from you in a coffee shop and reach my hand across the table to yours and tell you in person how much I want you to be whole and healed. I would love to look you in the eye and tell you that it is possible to have peace and joy, and deep, deep love and intimacy after cancer. I want to tell you these things because, though losing my breasts was incredibly painful (physically, emotionally, psychologically, and relationally), I have found healing. I have found peace. I have found joy. And I love my life in a way I didn't prior to January 20, 2016.

Dear friend, though cancer never really *goes away*, know this—life can still be good. So *very* good.

Appendix 1

Helpful Items for Recovery

1. *Mastectomy pillow(s)*—pillows that tuck into your armpit after surgery. They come in a variety of shapes and sizes, but their purpose is to alleviate pain and pressure after surgery. My mom and her friends make these, and you can request a set through a form at kimharms.net.

2. *Seatbelt cover*—a type of cushion that fits on your seatbelt to alleviate some of the discomfort of having a seatbelt up against your chest.

3. *Wedge pillow*—handy for recovering in bed, giving you the ability to sit in a reclined position instead of lying down flat.

4. *Recliner*—many women, including myself, find a recliner the most ideal place to recover. It allowed me to feel relatively comfortable and be in the living room so I didn't feel excluded from my family.

5. *Lanyard*—a must-have for showering with drains.

6. *Shirts with drain pockets*—available in a variety of options and styles. I wore a zipper-front hoodie with drain pockets sewn in. Some women prefer camisoles, a button-up shirt, or a Velcro shirt with drain pockets sewn in.

7. *Stool softeners*—prescription pain meds cause constipation. Be sure to use stool softeners to avoid the unpleasantness of not being able to poop.

8. *Comfy, easy on-and-off clothes*—button-down shirts, zipper hoodies, robes, elastic waist pants, etc. Any clothing that you find comfortable and easy to remove will make your life easier.

9. *Spray-on deodorant*—easier to spray on than to roll on when you have limited arm movement.

10. *ChapStick*—it's common to have dry, chapped lips after surgery.

11. *Nonskid slippers*—to keep your feet warm and prevent you from slipping on the floor.

12. *Extendable grabbers*—for the things you can't quite reach because of your limited mobility.

13. *Under-the-knee bolster pillow*—allows you to relax your legs while inhibiting them from stretching out and pulling at your abdomen after DIEP surgery.

14. *Shower chair*—if space in your shower allows, a shower chair makes the bathing experience more comfortable.

The History and the Law: The Development of Breast Re-construction and the Women's Health and Cancer Rights Act

"The more you know about the past, the better you are prepared for the future."
—Theodore Roosevelt

I am intrigued by how mastectomy and reconstruction procedures developed, and I'm thankful for all those who went before me and lobbied for laws that would be on my side as I endured the recon-struction process. This appendix is not an in-depth study of the law and history of mastectomy and breast reconstruction, but I'm hopeful you will find the information interesting and a worthwhile addition to your breast surgery arsenal.

I am beyond grateful my breast cancer diagnosis came in the twenty-first century. One hundred years earlier, chances are I wouldn't have made it out alive. I most definitely wouldn't be sporting *almost* normal-looking reconstructed breasts. But because millions of research dollars have been poured into finding better treatments and seeking cures over the past fifty years or so, I was told my chances of survival are 99 percent. I like those odds.

According to the National Cancer Institute (NCI), breast cancer far and away receives the most research funding out of all types of cancer.[1] Though breast cancer is still scary, this is good news for more than 266,000 women who will be diagnosed this year. And for the additional thousands of women who will test positive for a BRCA gene mutation, it's pretty good news too.

The significant amount of focus and funding for breast cancer research is in part due to the exposure given to the disease by the Susan G. Komen Foundation. You can hardly leave your house during the month of October (Breast Cancer Awareness Month) without seeing the Komen-inspired breast cancer pink. The foundation has raised more than 950 million dollars for research since its inception in 1982, and breast cancer mortality decreased 39 percent from 1989 to 2015.[2] That's a big deal.

As I've walked the breast cancer road and met many women who've also had the disease, I've been amazed at how treatment is precisely tailored to each individual's specific cancer diagnosis. Between different kinds of surgery, different chemotherapy cocktails, and hormone therapy and radiation, each woman diagnosed receives a protocol specific to her needs. It's a comfort to know how many options are out there in all forms of breast cancer treatment, but this book is about mastectomies and breast reconstruction, so I'll be focusing on the surgical side.

In the following outline, I'll give a brief overview of the history and law in regard to mastectomies and breast reconstruction. Surgical options are plentiful, and the end results are generally satisfactory. But this wasn't always the case.

The History of Mastectomy and Reconstruction

I. Early Breast Cancer Surgery

A. The first mastectomy was performed in 1889 by surgeon Dr. William Halstead. It was a radical mastectomy, which means that all of the breast tissue, lymph nodes, and underlying chest muscle were removed.

1. This aggressive surgery was believed by Halstead (a pioneer of breast surgery in his time) to be the best treatment for breast cancer.

2. It remained the most common surgery for breast cancer for nearly a century, despite challenges from other surgeons that less radical treatments could be successful in removing the cancerous tissue.[3]

a) Surgical treatment shifted to **lumpectomies** (breast conservation surgery) as evidence began to show radical mastectomy wasn't always necessary. A study in Guy's Hospital in London in the 1960s randomized patients who received radical mastectomies with those who received partial mastectomies and radiation. It found that breast-conserving surgery with radiation was a satisfactory means of removing early-stage breast cancers.[4]

b) A combination of lumpectomy and radiation is still a common treatment today for early-stage breast cancers.

II. Early Breast Reconstruction

A. Many early breast cancer surgeons opposed the idea of reconstructing the breast.

1. Halstead opposed any type of reconstruction because he believed it would "violate the local control of the disease."[5]

2. Others believed that reconstruction might hide a recurrence of the disease or unfavorably change the course of the disease.

a) A few surgeons attempted breast reconstruction surgery in the late 1800s and early 1900s despite strong resistance.

(1) Vincent Czerny, a professor of surgery at Heidelberg, is generally credited with the first autologous or flap breast reconstruction (when tissue is taken from another part of the woman's body and reassigned to the breast) in 1895 using a fist-sized lipoma (slow-growing fatty tissue) from the patient's flank (area between the ribs and hip.)[6]

(2) In 1905 and 1906, respectively, French surgeon Louis Ombrédanne and Italian surgeon Iginio Tansini are credited with performing the first pectoral muscle flap reconstruction and the first pedicled flap of skin and underlying latissimus dorsi muscle (broad flat muscle on each side of the back) reconstruction.[7]

In the early twentieth century, surgeons were on the right track. The world just wasn't ready yet. A variety of factors led breast reconstruction surgery to be a rarity in the first half of the twentieth century. These procedures often required multiple surgeries and caused significant scarring. The flaps often failed back then, making people resistant to undergo the surgery. These challenges, in addition to the influence of Halstead (who was adamantly opposed to reconstruction), kept reconstructive procedures from advancing until the 1960s.

III. Modern Breast Reconstruction

A. The modern era of breast reconstruction began in 1963 with the introduction of the silicone gel implant (invented by Thomas Cronin and Frank Gerow).[8]

1. This implant was placed under the remaining chest wall skin, either immediately after mastectomy or in a later surgery.

2. Concerns about the safety of silicone implants and fear of the silicone having a connection to a variety of diseases led the FDA to ban the use of silicone in implants in 1992.

3. In 2006, silicone implants were deemed safe and are again a common option in breast reconstruction.[9]

a) The first modern flap reconstructive surgery occurred in 1977.[10]

b) Skin expanders for breast reconstruction were introduced by plastic surgeon Chedomir Radovan in 1982.[11]

(1) Skin expanders allowed gradual expansion of skin to replace lost tissue from mastectomies.

(2) Though the technique has varied since it began, reconstruction with tissue expanders has become a common method to reconstruct a breast.

Breast reconstruction techniques continue to develop and change, but regardless of the technique, satisfactory results are pretty normal with modern procedures. Over the course of writing this book, I've spoken to many women who've chosen a variety of different reconstruction options, and the vast majority have been happy with the results of their reconstructive surgeries.

IV. Nipple Reconstruction

A. Nipple reconstruction became an option in the early 1980s.[12]

B. The most common approach to nipple reconstruction today utilizes the skin at the site where the new nipple will be located. A small incision is made, the new nipple is shaped, and then it's sutured to hold the form in place. Occasionally doctors take skin from the labia, inner thigh, or even the opposite breast, but those cases are the exception, not the norm.

The Law in Regard to Breast Cancer Surgeries

Two important pieces of legislation have passed in the past couple of decades—legislation that requires insurance providers to include reconstructive surgeries in their breast cancer coverage.

I. Women's Health and Cancer Rights Act

A. The Women's Health and Cancer Rights Act (WHCRA) was signed into law in 1998.[13] Prior to that year, breast reconstruction was considered cosmetic and not covered by insurance.

1. According to a study in the journal *Seminars in Plastic Surgery*, in the two decades preceding the passage of the WHCRA,

increasing research studies showed significant psychological and quality of life benefits for breast reconstruction.[14] Because of this, more and more medical professionals began considering it an important element of breast cancer recovery instead of simply a cosmetic procedure.

2. Many insurance providers still refused to add the coverage, steadfastly maintaining the cosmetic nature of the surgery. This is why legislation became necessary.

3. Under the WHCRA, in insurance packages that cover mastectomy, **benefits must include**: reconstruction of the breast removed by mastectomy, surgery to the opposite breast for symmetry purposes, an external prosthesis to be used before or during the reconstruction process, and coverage of any physical complications that arise from mastectomy.[15]

   a) The law doesn't apply to Medicaid and Medicare, but Medicare currently covers breast reconstruction if you had a mastectomy due to breast cancer. Medicaid coverage varies from state to state.

B. When the Affordable Care Act (ACA), or Obamacare, was signed into law in 2010, the provisions of the WHCRA stayed the same.[16] Health insurance plans that cover mastectomies still must also cover reconstruction under the new legislation. (See footer for resources where you can direct your questions regarding the WHCRA.)

II. Breast Cancer Patient Education Act

A. The Breast Cancer Patient Education Act (BCPEA) became law in 2015.[17]

   1. A report in the *Journal of the American Medical Association* states that almost one-fifth of women who do not undergo reconstruction lack knowledge about the available options.[18]

   2. By requiring insurance companies to inform each individual diagnosed with breast cancer of the services available to her, the law increases knowledge and puts more options in a woman's breast cancer treatment arsenal.

a) BCPEA became a reality with much help from the efforts of the American Society of Plastic Surgeons (ASPS).[19]

(1) Since 1998, insurance companies had been required to cover breast reconstruction after mastectomy, but they were not required to inform patients of reconstructive options.

(2) The ASPS believed this left a gap in access to reconstructive services due to a lack of patient knowledge.

(3) ASPS president David Song said, "In recent years, we have gained a deeper appreciation for the fact that cancer treatment leaves not just physical scars, but also psychological, spiritual and emotional scars. Reconstruction can play a role in treating those non-physical forms of pain, and all members of the cancer team have an obligation to, at a minimum, make sure that their patients understand their treatment options. Anything less is unacceptable."[20]

I don't know about you, but I'm pretty grateful countless people fought for the rights of breast cancer patients so that my treatment could be top-notch. A breast cancer diagnosis will never be a happy thing. None of us wanted to hear the words "You have cancer." But because of the efforts of so many women and concerned medical professionals who have gone before us, we are able to walk into breast cancer with an arsenal of highly successful treatment options.

Questions or concerns about this law can be directed to the following places:

- *The US Department of Labor*: WHCRA information can be accessed on their website at https://www.dol.gov/agencies/ebsa/laws-and-regulations/laws/whcra. Or you can call their toll-free number: 1-866-487-2365.
- *The Employee Benefits Security Administration*: a special office of the Department of Labor. Call 1-866-444-3272 for information about employer-based health insurance.

- *Your health plan administrator*: a number should be listed on your insurance card.
- *Your state insurance commissioner's office*: the number should be listed in your local phone book in the state government section, or you can find it at the National Association of Insurance Commissioners online at www.naic.org/state_web_map.htm. If you can't find the number elsewhere, call 1-866-470-NAIC (1-866-470-6242).[21]

Resources

1. "Funding for Research Areas." National Cancer Institute, December 20, 2018. https://www.cancer.gov/about-nci/budget/fact-book/data/research-funding.

2. "How Our Research Is Making a Difference." Susan G. Komen Foundation, accessed December 3, 2019. https://ww5.komen.org/WhatWeDo/WeFundResearch/ResearchAccomplishments/ResearchAccomplishments.html.

3. Chintamani. 2013. "The Paradigm Shifts in the Management of Breast Cancer: Have We Finally Arrived?" *Indian Journal of Surgery* 75, no. 6: 419–23. https://www.ncbi.nlm.nih.gov/pmc/articles/PMC3900753/.

4. Uroski, Theodore W., Jr., and Colen, Lawrence B. "History of Breast Reconstruction." *Seminars in Plastic Surgery* 18, no. 2: 65–69. https://www.ncbi.nlm.nih.gov/pmc/articles/PMC2884724/.

5. Ibid.

6. Hultman, Charles Scott. 2002. "Perforator Flap Breast Reconstruction." *Breast Disease* 16, no. 1: 93–106.

7. Uroski and Colen, "History of Breast Reconstruction."

8. O'Leary, Naomi; Cutler, David; and Sage, Alexandria. "Timeline: A Short History of Breast Implants." Reuters, January 26, 2012. https://www.reuters.com/article/us-france-implants-pip-idUSTRE80P12V20120126.

9. Ibid.

10. Uroski and Colen, "History of Breast Reconstruction."

11. Ibid.

12. Ibid.

13. "Women's Health and Cancer Rights Act." American Cancer Society, updated May 13, 2019. https://www.cancer.org/treatment/finding-and-paying-for-treatment/understanding-health-insurance/health-insurance-laws/womens-health-and-cancer-rights-act.html.

14. Wilkins, Edwin G., and Alderman, Amy K. 2004. "Breast Reconstruction Practices in North America: Current Trends and Future Priorities." *Seminars in Plastic Surgery* 18, no. 2: 149–55. https://www.ncbi.nlm.nih.gov/pmc/articles/PMC2884720/.

15. "Women's Health and Cancer Rights Act."

16. Ibid.

17. "ASPS Secures Passage of the Breast Cancer Patient Education Act." American Society of Plastic Surgeons, December 18, 2015. https://www.plasticsurgery.org/news/press-releases/asps-secures-passage-of-the-breast-cancer-patient-education-act.

18. Ibid.

19. Ibid.
20. Ibid.
21. O'Leary et al., "Timeline: A Short History of Breast Implants."

Glossary

The definitions included in this glossary were collected and modified from a variety of sources, including: Aesthetic Plastic Surgery, PC (https://www.aestheticplasticsurgerypc.com/), American Cancer Society (https://www.cancer.org/), American College of Surgeons (https://www.facs.org/), American Society of Plastic Surgeons (https://www.plasticsurgery.org), BreastCancer.org (https://www.breastcancer.org/), the Food and Drug Administration (FDA) (https://www.fda.gov/media/80685/download), *Frankly Speaking About Breast Cancer: Spotlight on Breast Reconstruction* (https://www.cancersupport-community.org/sites/default/files/d7/document/fsac_spotlight_on_breast_reconstruction.pdf), The National Cancer Institute (https://www.cancer.gov/), and the input of Susan L. Beck, DO.

autologous tissue flap reconstruction: flap surgeries move healthy tissue from the abdomen to the breast. There are three types: the **DIEP (deep inferior epigastric artery perforator) flap**, **latissimus flap**, and **TRAM (transverse rectus abdominis muscle) flap**.

acellular dermal matrix: human tissue used for support and stabilization of the breast expander or implant. It's incorporated into the surrounding tissue within three weeks.

aestheticist: a medical tattoo artist.

bilateral (double) mastectomy: a surgery to remove the tissue of both breasts.

BRCA1 and BRCA2: genes which, when damaged (mutated), place a woman at greater risk of developing breast cancer and/or ovarian cancer compared with women who do not have this mutation. Men can also carry the gene mutation.

breast augmentation (boob job): utilizes implants or fat to enhance the size and shape of already-existing breasts. The woman's natural breast tissue remains intact, and an implant is added to the breast tissue for aesthetic reasons. This procedure is completed using a small incision in an inconspicuous area, like the armpit or the underside of the areola.

breast reconstruction: the rebuilding of breasts after a mastectomy.

capsular contracture: when an unusually large tissue capsule that forms around the breast implant squeezes the implant. This can cause pain and distort the shape of the breast.

delayed reconstruction: when a woman chooses to wait months, or even years, after mastectomy to have her breasts reconstructed.

DIEP (deep inferior epigastric artery perforator) flap: a procedure that uses fat and skin from the abdomen, leaving the muscle intact, to create a breast mound. This is a free flap surgery ("free" because the tissue is completely severed from the abdominal wall and moved) followed by the reattachment of blood vessels.

direct-to-implant reconstruction: reconstruction completed at the time of the mastectomy. It can be done by placing the implant underneath or above the chest muscle. Donated cadaver tissue (**acellular dermal matrix**) or an absorbable mesh is inserted in the shape of a sling to hold the implant in place.

dog ears: pockets of fat under the arms after mastectomy. This more commonly occurs in women who choose to go flat.

Doppler probe (Doppler blood flow) monitor: an implantable ultrasound probe attached to a wire leading from the reattached blood vessels to the outside of the body, where it is connected to a monitor that keeps track of blood flow.

drain bulbs: a bulb-shaped container attached to tubing that is inserted into the body after a surgical procedure. The bulb collects fluid that drains from the body after surgery.

ductal carcinoma in situ (DCIS): a highly curable, non-invasive form of breast cancer that consists of cancer cells localized to the breast ducts. Also called stage 0.

expansion appointment: an appointment where the plastic surgeon uses a long needle attached to a syringe filled with saline to increase the size of the tissue expander. (Silicone is not used during the expansion process. It is only an option for permanent implants.) This allows the breast skin (and sometimes muscle, depending on final implant placement) to slowly stretch over a period of time until the breast reaches the desired size.

exchange surgery: the second stage of two-stage breast reconstruction surgery (generally outpatient) in which the expander is removed and replaced with a permanent implant. This surgery is significantly shorter and less invasive than the first phase (mastectomy and expander insertion reconstruction surgery) but does require a couple of weeks to heal.

fat transfer: a procedure that uses a person's own fat to fill in irregularities.

flap reconstruction: a procedure where tissue is taken from another part of the woman's body and reassigned to the breast. Skin, muscle, and fat tissue can all be used. Several places on the body can be used as donor sites for flap reconstruction, but the two most common sites are the abdomen and upper back.

free TRAM flap: in this procedure, tissue and muscle (but usually less muscle than the **pedicled TRAM flap**) are completely severed and moved to the chest, where the blood vessels are then reattached. This procedure takes longer than the TRAM flap because of the time needed to reattach blood vessels, but there is less risk of losing abdominal strength in this procedure.

gluteal free flap: uses tissue from the buttocks and is similar to the **free TRAM flap** in that the tissue is cut out and moved to the chest where the blood vessels are reattached.

going flat: a term used when a woman chooses not to undergo reconstruction after a mastectomy.

guided meditation: meditation in response to someone else through a variety of possible means, like in person, video, audio, or written text.

gummy bear implants: utilizes a semi-solid silicone gel that holds its form even if the implant breaks. Because of the thickness of the gel, these implants feel less like natural breast tissue than regular silicone, but they don't risk leaking if the implant is punctured.

hematoma: a blood clot that forms in the tissues outside of the blood vessel.

hormone therapy: a type of cancer treatment for hormone receptor–positive cancers. These hormonal drugs keep estrogen and progesterone from attaching to the receptors on breast cancer cells.

implant: a silicone gel–filled or saline-filled flexible sac inserted either above or underneath the pectoral muscle in breast reconstruction and cosmetic breast surgery.

implant reconstruction: a surgery in which the breast(s) is rebuilt using a silicone or saline implant that can be placed under or over the pectoral muscle.

immediate reconstruction: see **direct-to-implant reconstruction**.

invasive ductal carcinoma: cancer that originates in the milk ducts. Accounts for about 80 percent of all breast cancer diagnoses.

invasive lobular carcinoma: cancer that originates in the milk-producing glands (lobules).

latissimus dorsi flap reconstruction: a tunneling procedure like the **pedicled TRAM flap**, but it takes tissue from the upper back, tunneling it under the skin to the chest to make a pocket for an implant.

lollipop lift: a breast lift performed by creating an incision around the areola and another incision vertically from the areola to the breast crease, creating a "lollipop" shape.

lumpectomy: a surgery which removes a tumor and a small amount of tissue surrounding it (a **margin**) but does not remove the whole breast.

margin: the edge or border of the tissue removed in cancer surgery. The margin is described as "negative" or "clean" when the pathologist finds no cancer cells at the edge of the tissue, suggesting that all of the cancer has been removed.

nipple-sparing mastectomy: a procedure that removes the breast tissue while preserving the nipple and areola.

non-abdominal flap reconstruction: a surgery that moves healthy tissue from the upper back, buttocks, or inner thigh to the breast area. These surgeries include the **latissimus dorsi flap**, the **gluteal artery perforator (GAP) free flap**, and the **transverse upper gracilis (TUG) flap**.

ON-Q pain pump: a type of pain relief system that utilizes a pump ball connected to a tube, inserted at the surgical site, that continuously delivers local anesthesia to block the pain in the area of the procedure.

oophorectomy: surgical removal of one or both ovaries.

pedicled (attached) TRAM flap: a procedure where the rectus abdominal muscle is tunneled underneath the skin of the abdomen to the reconstruction site, allowing the muscle to remain connected to its original blood supply. These are sometimes called "muscle-transfer flaps" because most or all of the rectus abdominal muscle is used.

prosthesis: a breast form made to mimic a natural breast, insertable into your bra.

previvor: a woman who undergoes a bilateral mastectomy prior to a cancer diagnosis due to testing positive for a mutation on their BRCA1 or BRCA2 gene (which greatly increases future risk of breast cancer).

prophylactic bilateral mastectomy: a mastectomy performed prior to a cancer diagnosis.

round implants: circular-shaped implants in the breast. These are the most commonly used implants in breast augmentation because of the fullness they give the breast and because the implant can rotate within the pocket without changing the contour of the breast.

saline implants: breast implants filled with saline (salt water) solution. They tend to be less malleable than silicone implants, but in the case of a punctured implant the body can naturally absorb the liquid, unlike silicone.

sentinel lymph node: the first lymph node to which cancer will spread from the original tumor site.

silicone implants: breast implants filled with a silicone gel. Fears about the silicone leaking into the body in the event of a puncture led the FDA to research the safety of these implants in the 1990s. *They were deemed safe and have been in use ever since the completion of that study in 2006.*

smooth implants: can move around within the implant pocket, acting more like a natural breast. They can cause a visible rippling under the skin.

survivor: from the time of receiving a breast cancer diagnosis until death, a person is considered a survivor.

teardrop implants: shaped similarly to the natural breast, with more silicone or saline along the base of the breast than the top. The biggest risk with this type of implant is that if it rotates out of place, it will change the contour of the breast.

textured implants[*]: can stick to scar tissue, limiting their movement in the breast pocket. These implants are less likely to get repositioned, but they also move less naturally.

tissue expander: a balloon-like temporary implant that is gradually inflated with a saline solution to stretch skin (and sometimes muscle) to make room for the permanent implant.

tissue flap reconstruction: procedures that use tissue from the abdomen, back, thighs, or buttocks to rebuild the breast.

triple negative breast cancer: an aggressive form of breast cancer whose cells test negative for estrogen, progesterone, and HER2—three things that drive the growth of common breast cancers. Because of this, it doesn't respond to common treatment options used for other breast cancer types. More likely to occur in pre-menopausal African-American women.

TUG (transverse upper gracilis) flap: a procedure that takes tissue extending from the lower buttocks to the inner thigh. Good candidates for this procedure are women whose thighs touch. Like the abdominal flap surgeries, this is a less likely option for thin women.

two-stage reconstruction: during the first stage, a mastectomy is performed followed by the placement of an expander (either under or over the chest muscle). Prior to the second stage, several expansion appointments occur. The second stage, where the expander is replaced by a permanent implant, generally occurs months after the first stage.

unilateral (single) mastectomy: a surgery to remove the tissue of one breast.

---

[*] Note: Allergan BIOCELL Textured Breast Implants were recalled in July 2019 due to a link to implant-associated large cell lymphoma.

Recommended Resources

Print

Battlefield of the Mind: Winning the Battle in Your Mind (Warner Faith, 2002) by Joyce Meyer

Better Than New: Insider Tips from a Glamour Girl on Surviving Breast Cancer, Mastectomy, and Reconstruction (Two Harbors Press, 2011) by Sally Barnes

Breast Cancer Husband: How to Help Your Wife (And Yourself) Through Diagnosis, Treatment and Beyond (Rodale Books, 2004) by Marc Silver

Breast Cancer Surgery and Reconstruction: What's Right for You (Rowman and Littlefield, 2016) by Patricia Anstett and Kathleen Galligan

Breasts: The Owner's Manual: Every Woman's Guide to Reducing Cancer Risk, Making Treatment Choices, and Optimizing Outcomes (Thomas Nelson, 2018) by Dr. Kristi Funk

The Breast Reconstruction Guidebook (Fourth Edition): Issues and Answers from Research to Recovery (Johns Hopkins University Press, 2017) by Kathy Steligo

Dr. Susan Love's Breast Book (Sixth Edition) (DeCapo Lifelong Books, 2015) by Dr. Susan M. Love

Guide to Breast Reconstruction After Mastectomy: What to Do After You Are Diagnosed (CreateSpace, 2015) by Dr. Ben J. Childers

Self-Advocacy: A Cancer Survivor's Handbook (National Coalition for Cancer Survivorship, 2009) compiled by Susan L. Scherr, https://canceradvocacy.org/wp-content/uploads/2013/01/Self_Advocacy.pdf

Ticking Off Breast Cancer (Hashtag Press, 2019) by Sara Liyanage

Warrior in Pink: A Story of Cancer, Community, and the God Who Comforts (Discovery House, 2014) by Vivian Mabuni

Online

American Cancer Society: https://www.cancer.org/

American Society of Plastic Surgeons: https://www.plasticsurgery.org/

Authentic Intimacy: https://www.authenticintimacy.com/

BCHealthline: https://www.instagram.com/bchealthline/

BreastCancer.org: https://www.breastcancer.org/

Breast Cancer Wellness Magazine: http://www.breastcancerwellness.org/

BreastReconstruction.org: http://breastreconstruction.org/

Cleaning for a Reason: https://cleaningforareason.org/

DiepCjourney: https://diepcjourney.com/

DJ Breast Cancer: https://www.djbreastcancer.org/

Facing Our Risk of Cancer Empowered (FORCE): https://www.facingour-risk.org/

Flat & Fabulous: https://www.flatandfabulous.org/

Functional Rehab After Breast Cancer: https://www.uhn.ca/PatientsFamilies/Health_Information/Health_Topics/Documents/Your_Functional_Rehabilitation_After_Breast_Surgery.pdf

Hidden Scar Breast Cancer Surgery: https://breastcancersurgery.com/

Life Reconstructed (my personal website with blog and resources): http://kimharms.net/

Living Beyond Breast Cancer: https://www.lbbc.org/

Sunnybrook Health Sciences Centre: https://sunnybrook.ca/content/?page=mastectomy-exercises-after-surgery

Susan G. Komen Foundation: https://www.komen.org/

Verywell Health: https://www.verywellhealth.com/arm-exercises-after-breast-surgery-430189

Wildfire Magazine: https://www.wildfirecommunity.org/

ABOUT THE AUTHOR

Kim Harms is a graduate of Iowa State University with a BA in English and an emphasis in journalism. A freelance writer and breast cancer survivor, she lives in Huxley, Iowa, with her husband and three sons and is widely published in magazines, newspapers, and devotionals.

ABOUT FAMILIUS

VISIT OUR WEBSITE: WWW.FAMILIUS.COM

Familius is a global trade publishing company that publishes books and other content to help families be happy. We believe that the family is the fundamental unit of society and that happy families are the foundation of a happy life. We recognize that every family looks different, and we passionately believe in helping all families find greater joy. To that end, we publish books for children and adults that invite families to live the Familius Ten Habits of Happy Families: *love together, play together, learn together, work together, talk together, heal together, read together, eat together, give together,* and *laugh together.* Founded in 2012, Familius is located in Sanger, California.

CONNECT

Facebook: www.facebook.com/familiustalk
Twitter: @familiustalk, @paterfamilius1
Pinterest: www.pinterest.com/familius
Instagram: @familiustalk

FAMILIUS

*The most important work you ever do will be
within the walls of your own home.*